Contributors

Rebecca Harmon, MPM, RHIA
Deyal Donna Riley, CHI, CPT
Jahangir Moini, M.D., M.P.H., C.Ph.T.
Contributing Writers

Candice Bennett, MT (ASCP)
Contributing Reviewer

Kelly Von Lunen, BS Journalism
Michelle Renner, BS Journalism
Editors

Mandy Tallmadge, BS Communication
Design Associate

Christine Bush, BS Communications
Morgan Smith, BS Broadcast Journalism
Media Developers

Sharif Wilson, BA Scientific and Technical Arts
Graphic Designer

Printed in October 2012.

INTELLECTUAL PROPERTY NOTICE

IMPORTANT NOTICE TO THE READER

Table of Contents

Processing

Safety and Compliance Considerations

Case Studies

Summary

References

>>INTRODUCTION

Learning Objectives
After reading this study guide, you will be able to:

- *Positively identify the patient.*

- *Ensure patient safety throughout the collection process.*

- *Recognize common complications from primary collection, such as lack of blood flow, hematoma, petechiae, and nerve injury.*

- *Prepare peripheral blood smears.*

- *Calculate volume requirements to avoid causing iatrogenic anemia.*

- *Perform order of draw when performing venipuncture and capillary collection.*

- *Label all specimens.*

- *Assist other health care professionals with blood culture collections.*

- *Collect blood samples for inborn errors of metabolism, such as PKU and galactosemia.*

- *Follow exposure control plans in the event of an occupational exposure.*

- *Adhere to regulations regarding workplace safety, such as OSHA and NIOSH regulations.*

Overview

Certified Phlebotomy Technician (CPT) is a certification the National Healthcareer Association (NHA) issues to a person who passes a national certification exam. CPTs work in a variety of clinical settings, including hospitals and physicians' offices. The CPT certification can lead to additional employment opportunities in the health care field and provide a foundation for future training. In many areas of the country and in many health care facilities, finding employment as a phlebotomy technician, earning a higher salary, and advancing in the field cannot be done without a phlebotomy technician certification.

The purpose of the CPT certification is to establish a standard of care among phlebotomy technicians. In order to sit for the CPT examination, the applicant must have a high school diploma or GED and complete an approved training program.

The CPT exam consists of 110 multiple-choice questions, with 100 of those items being scored. If your school is a registered NHA test site, you may take a proctored exam via computer or in paper-pencil format. You also have the option to take the exam via computer at a PSI testing center. You are allotted 110 minutes to complete the exam. You must achieve a scaled score of 390 out of 500 to pass the exam. Exam scores are sent to your home address about 3 to 5 business days after NHA receives your completed answer sheet.

This study guide provides students with the information they need to successfully take the CPT exam. This guide is intended to help students feel comfortable and confident when taking the certification exam. Memorizing facts is necessary, but that is just the first step in learning. Understanding the background and scientific rationales behind the information is not only the best way to truly grasp the material, but also offers the greatest chance for successfully passing the exam.

Each chapter of this study guide begins with a list of learning objectives that introduces the concepts contained within the chapter. The key instructional content, or body of each chapter, follows the CPT test plan, which can be found before the first chapter. Following the key instructional content, you will find a chapter summary, which recaps the main points within the chapter; drill questions, which assess your knowledge of the chapter subjects; and a terms and definitions section, which defines the bolded words within the chapter.

Chapter 1: Patient Preparation

Chapter 1 provides you with an understanding of the basic patient preparation necessary prior to performing a phlebotomy procedure. Learning these steps is critical to becoming a CPT, as they give you a solid beginning on which to build your knowledge in the subsequent chapters.

Chapter 2: Collection Techniques

The second chapter is split into two sections: primary collections and special collections. The primary collections section prepares you for basic blood collection through venipuncture and dermal punctures of the finger or heel. You will learn the proper techniques for safely and correctly obtaining quality specimens from patients who need testing performed. Accurately collecting specimens helps physicians and nurses provide the best care for patients. As a CPT, you'll contribute to high-quality health care delivery when performing duties in a safe and accurate manner. The special collections section reviews when you'll need to collect special types of specimens to meet patient needs. This section also reviews the most common special collection practices and prepares you to safely and appropriately collect and process them.

Chapter 3: Processing

Next, Chapter 3 lists and describes the many tasks of processing patient specimens after collection. After proper collection, careful handling and processing are most important steps to ensure that the test results are timely and accurate and serve the best interest of the patients.

Chapter 4: Safety and Compliance Considerations

Chapter 4 goes over important safety and compliance guidelines to keep in mind when working with patients, their protected health information, and potentially infectious materials. CPTs must learn to work safely, protecting the health and safety or their patients, as well as themselves and fellow health care workers. They must follow laws and regulations in place to protect patients' privacy and the security of patient information, and to remain ready to assist when patient emergencies arise.

Case Studies

Following the chapters, there are three scenarios that test your accumulated knowledge in all areas of the study guide. Each scenario represents a real-life situation and requires critical thinking skills to effectively complete the discussion questions that follow.

NHA Certified Phlebotomy Technician (CPT)
2011 Detailed Test Plan
100 scored items, 10 pretest items

		# scored items
1.	**Patient Preparation**	**23**
	A. Conduct appropriate introduction to the patient.	
	B. Explain the phlebotomy procedure to be performed to the patient.	
	C. Review the requisition for testing requirements and patient identity.	
	D. Receive implied or informed consent from the patient.	
	E. Positively identify the patient.	
	F. Determine appropriate site for sample requirement.	
	G. Select a site that minimizes patient risk.	
	H. Determine venipuncture site accessibility based on patient age and condition.	
	I. Apply appropriate antiseptic agent using aseptic technique.	
	J. Verify patient compliance with testing requirements (e.g., fasting, medication, basal state).	
2.	**Collection Techniques**	**40**
	A. Primary Collections	30
	1. Demonstrate proper insertion and removal techniques for venipuncture.	
	2. Perform capillary collection method based on patient age and condition.	
	3. Ensure patient safety throughout the collection process.	
	4. Perform venipuncture steps in correct order (e.g., evacuated tube system, syringe, winged collection set).	
	5. Perform capillary (dermal) puncture steps in correct order.	
	6. Recognize common complications from primary collection (e.g., lack of blood flow, hematoma, petechiae, nerve injury).	
	7. Identify problematic patient signs and symptoms throughout collection (e.g., syncope, diaphoresis, nausea, seizure).	

NHA Certified Phlebotomy Technician (CPT)
2011 Detailed Test Plan
100 scored items, 10 pretest items

	# scored items
8. Follow order of draw when performing venipuncture.	
9. Follow order of draw when performing capillary collection.	
10. Ensure that tube additives are appropriate for testing requirements.	
11. Assemble equipment needed for primary blood collections.	
12. Invert evacuated tubes with additives after collection.	
13. Verify quality of equipment (e.g., sterility, expiration date, manufacturer's defects).	
B. Special Collections	**10**
1. Prepare peripheral blood smears.	
2. Perform blood culture collections.	
3. Assist other health care professionals with blood culture collections.	
4. Collect blood samples for inborn errors of metabolism (e.g., PKU, galactosemia).	
5. Perform phlebotomy for blood donations.	
6. Calculate volume requirements to avoid causing iatrogenic anemia.	
3. Processing	**27**
A. Label all specimens.	
B. Perform quality control for CLIA-waived procedures.	
C. Transport specimens based on handling requirements (e.g., temperature, light, time).	
D. Explain non-blood specimen collection procedures to patients (e.g., stool, urine, semen, sputum).	
E. Handle patient-collected, non-blood specimens.	
F. Avoid pre-analytical errors when collecting blood specimens (e.g., QNS, hemolysis).	

NHA Certified Phlebotomy Technician (CPT) 2011 Detailed Test Plan 100 scored items, 10 pretest items	# scored items
G. Adhere to chain of custody guidelines when required (e.g., forensic studies, blood alcohol, drug screen).	
H. Prepare samples for transportation to a reference (outside) laboratory.	
I. Coordinate communication between non-laboratory personnel for processing and collection.	
J. Use technology to input and retrieve specimen data.	
K. Report critical values for point of care testing.	
L. Distribute laboratory results to ordering providers.	
4. Safety and Compliance Considerations	10
A. Adhere to regulations regarding workplace safety (e.g., OSHA, NIOSH).	
B. Adhere to regulations regarding operational standards (e.g., JCAHO, CLSI).	
C. Adhere to HIPAA regulations regarding protected health information (PHI).	
D. Follow exposure control plans in the event of occupational exposure.	
E. Follow transmission-based precautions (e.g., iatrogenic, airborne, droplet, contact).	
F. Wear personal protective equipment while following standard precautions (e.g., gloves, gowns, masks, shoe covers).	
G. Sanitize hands to prevent the spread of infections.	
H. Initiate first aid when necessary.	
I. Initiate CPR when necessary.	

01 >> PATIENT PREPARATION

Learning Objectives

At the end of this chapter, you will be able to:

- *Conduct an appropriate introduction to the patient.*

- *Explain the phlebotomy procedure to be performed to the patient.*

- *Review the requisition form for testing requirements and patient identity.*

- *Receive implied or informed consent from the patient.*

- *Positively identify the patient.*

- *Determine appropriate site for sample requirements.*

- *Select a site that minimizes patient risk.*

- *Determine venipuncture site accessibility based on patient's age and condition.*

- *Apply appropriate antiseptic agent using aseptic technique.*

- *Verify patient compliance with testing requirements (e.g., fasting, medication, basal state).*

Overview

The blood collection procedure begins with reviewing the requisition form before approaching the patient. This review assists in determining whether the documentation is correct and helps establish the priority of the patient's tests. The procedure continues with the preparation of the patient. As a phlebotomy technician, you must properly introduce yourself to the patient. Positive identification of patients is essential before performing any medical procedure. Failing to positively identify a patient may result in misdiagnosis or incorrect treatment. Evaluate a patient's ability to understand the procedure that you will perform. Then, educate the patient on the risks and complications and what they must do if these issues occur. Obtain patient consent before beginning any procedure. Evaluate patients as to age and condition to determine which site would be appropriate for blood collection. Choose a site for blood collection that minimizes risk to the patient and also has the best chance for a successful blood collection. Use the proper antiseptic agent to cleanse the site before blood collection.

Ensure that the patient has performed any necessary preparation prior to performing the blood collection.

Conduct Appropriate Introduction to the Patient

The phlebotomist is often the first clinical person patients interact with when they arrive at a health care facility. As a phlebotomist, you may be the first person to perform a medical procedure or test on the patient. Therefore, it is very important to look at patients as individuals, and interact with them on their level. Although many patients will be sitting in your chair for routine blood testing, others may be facing a surgery or may be processing bad news in the form of a life-altering diagnosis. The best phlebotomists not only accurately withdraw blood from their patients' veins, but they also handle each patient with respect, individual attention, and professionalism.

Before beginning a blood collection procedure, it is important to let the patient know who you are and what procedure you will perform. State your first name to the patient; last name is not necessary. Inform the patient that you are a phlebotomy technician and that you are going to collect a blood sample. Wear an identification badge that is visible to the patient. If you are a student, let the patient know. Always introduce yourself, even if you have drawn blood from the patient before. Always tell the patient what you are going to do.

Explain the Phlebotomy Procedure to the Patient

Patient education about the phlebotomy process is straightforward and easy to integrate into the procedure. Tell the patient what is going to happen, why it is being done, and what to do if there are any problems during the procedure. Lastly, explain what complications can occur after the procedure, as well as what to do if complications happen.

Ask the patient whether he has ever had blood drawn. If the answer is yes, ask him whether he has any questions, and answer any questions that he may have. Do not use technical language or medical jargon when explaining the phlebotomy procedure to him. Try to use familiar terms.

If the patient has never had blood drawn, explain the procedure by following these steps:

- Discuss the steps of the procedure: examination and preparation of a site, application of a tourniquet, insertion of the needle, filling the blood tubes, and applying a bandage to the venipuncture site after you obtain the blood and the needle is removed.

- Advise the patient that he will experience a slight bit of pain when the needle is inserted and while the tubes are being filled. Never tell the patient "This won't hurt," because that is not true; venipuncture may hurt.

- Tell the patient to say something immediately if he experiences severe pain or feels sick.

- Inform the patient about the complications of venipuncture, such as excessive bruising, hematoma, infection, prolonged bleeding, or serious pain. Then tell the patient what to do if these should occur. It is best to do this after the venipuncture process is complete.

The complications include:

- Excessive bleeding: A small amount of bleeding after a venipuncture is common. There is no precise definition of excessive bleeding. However, a reasonable rule of thumb is that if the small gauze pad used to cover the venipuncture site becomes completely soaked with blood, the patient should return to the laboratory or ask a physician or nurse for help.

- Severe pain: The patient should seek help if he has severe pain after a venipuncture, or if the pain from the venipuncture lasts more than a few minutes.

- Lack of sensation: Instruct the patient to immediately return to the laboratory or immediately ask a physician or nurse for help if there is numbness or tingling in the arm that was used for a venipuncture. The numbness or tingling should last only a few hours. Otherwise, the potential for nerve damage could occur.

- Excessive bruising: As with bleeding and pain, a slight amount of bruising at the venipuncture site is normal. However, if the bruising spreads over a large area, this indicates the venipuncture site is still bleeding. There is no definition of the size of bruise that is excessive, but a reasonable rule of thumb is to define a hematoma as greater in diameter than the gauze pad.

- Infection: If the area around the site of a venipuncture becomes red, swollen and painful, there may be an infection present. Hematomas can become infected, as well. Patients should see a physician if this occurs.

- Patient feels unwell: Patients who need blood tests often have an ongoing illness or a chronic medical condition, and they can develop signs or symptoms as a reaction to a venipuncture.

After speaking with your patient about excessive bleeding, bruising, and pain, inform him that if he feels sick in any way, he should return to the laboratory or ask a physician or a nurse for help. Also provide an opportunity for the patient to ask any questions that he may have, and answer any questions promptly.

Review the Requisition for Testing Requirements and Patient Identity

Physicians, physician's assistants, and, in some circumstances, nurse practitioners may order laboratory tests. Do not accept an order from any other health care professional. The laboratory order form, also known as a **requisition form**, should have at least the following information: patient's full name, patient's date of birth, patient's Social Security number (or other identifying number such as medical record number), patient's gender, name of the tests, and name of

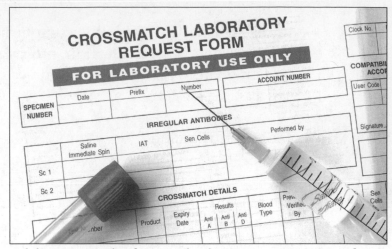

A laboratory order form is also known as a requisition form.

the person ordering the test. In addition, there should be space on the form for the phlebotomy technician to document when the blood sample was obtained. Examine the requisition form to verify the requested tests and the appropriate times to collect them. Verify whether there are any special preparations or restrictions that must occur prior to the collection, such as patient fasting or basal state. It is also important to determine the priority of the blood collection. The terms **stat**, medical emergency, and **ASAP** indicate that physicians or others need the test results right away, so you must collect the blood specimens as soon as it is safely possible. A routine blood collection is important to a patient's diagnosis and treatment, but it does not indicate any urgency. If any information is missing, return the requisition form to the provider for clarification before performing the blood collection.

Specimen labels should accompany the requisition form. These are sticky labels with the patient's identifying information printed on them. You will then place the labels on the blood samples. If no labels are available, you should write the patient's last name, first name, date of birth or other specific identifier (this will depend on your facility policy), the date and time the specimen was collected, and your initials. All identification labeling should be done before leaving the patient's bedside.

Receive Implied or Informed Consent from the Patient

Before performing a blood collection on a patient, it is essential to obtain the patient's consent. There are different types of consent, including expressed, informed, implied, and consent for minors. There is also the refusal of consent.

- Expressed consent: May be given verbally or in writing, and is essential for high-risk procedures. It also will be used for surgery and in medical research.

- Informed consent: Requires that a patient be provided with information in a language the patient can understand.

- Implied consent: When the patient's actions imply that he is giving consent to the procedure. (Example: A phlebotomist enters a patient's room and the patient extends his arm.) This form of consent may be necessary in emergency medical situations.

- Consent for minors: In most cases, the parent or guardian must give consent for procedures you will perform on a minor.

- Refusal of consent: Any patient may refuse to grant consent for any reason. Whether for personal choice, religious, or other reasons, a patient has a right to refuse. When a patient does refuse, in most cases, you need to obtain written proof of this refusal to protect both the phlebotomist and patient. The person who ordered the test must be informed of the refusal.

Positively Identify the Patient

Proper patient identification is the most important step to ensure that tests are performed on the correct patient. Correctly identifying a patient should involve at least two of the following actions:

- Ask the patient to state and spell her full name.

- Ask the patient for her date of birth.

- Ask the patient for the last four digits of her Social Security number (if the medical facility policy requires this information). Some outpatient facilities may ask for photo identification to be shown (e.g., a student or work ID, driver's license or passport).

This information needs to be compared to the name, date of birth, and Social Security number or **medical identification number** on the patient's wristband for inpatients – outpatients often do not have a wristband – and the laboratory order form. If there are any discrepancies, do not perform the phlebotomy procedure. Always ask the patient for her personal information. Never state a patient's personal information and then wait for her to confirm that the information is correct. A patient may be unable to provide her name and identifying information because of unconsciousness, speaking challenges (e.g., a patient who is using a mechanical ventilator), or because of a language barrier. In situations such as these, the patient's wristband and someone who knows the patient – someone whose identity you can verify, such as the nurse, spouse, or patient's guardian – should positively identify the patient. Use an interpreter to assist with patients who speak another language. Always check the medical facility's protocol if you are unsure how to properly identify patients who cannot do so themselves, or are not legally able to do so (as with children).

Patients may wonder why you are asking so many questions. Reassure them by explaining that the questions are intentional and help to ensure accurate test results.

Once you've identified the patient correctly, you may perform the phlebotomy. However, you should never perform a venipuncture if:

- The patient does not have an identification wristband. (If in an inpatient, surgical, or rehab facility, ask the patient's nurse to place a wristband on the patient before the procedure.)

- There are any discrepancies between the order forms, the personal information the patient provides, or the patient's identification wristband.

- The patient cannot identify herself, and there is no one who can identify the patient.

Determining the Appropriate Site for Sample Requirement

Minimizing complications and safely performing the venipuncture requires that you correctly choose and prepare the site for venipuncture. There are three basic categories of blood vessels: arteries, capillaries, and veins. When performing venipuncture, you access the veins.

The three veins present in the antecubital fossa that you will use for phlebotomy are the following:

- Median cubital vein: This vein is often the first choice of phlebotomy technicians. It lies in the center or near the center of the antecubital fossa. It is a large vein, and it does not usually move when you puncture it. In some patients (especially patients who are obese), the median cubital vein may not be visible, but you can often find it by palpating.

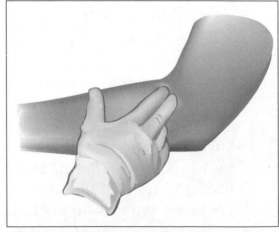

Palpating helps to identify the best vein for the venipuncture procedure.

- Cephalic vein: The cephalic vein is usually the second choice of phlebotomy technicians. The cephalic vein lies in the antecubital fossa on the lateral aspect of the forearm. (Note: Lateral means toward the side, away from the center of the body.) It is a large vein, and although you can easily palpate it, it is not usually visible. It tends to roll and can be difficult to stabilize. This is a vein that often can be palpated, even in obese patients.

- Brachial vein: The brachial vein should be the last choice when selecting a site. The brachial vein lies in the antecubital fossa on the medial aspect of the forearm. (Note: Medial means toward the middle, close to the center of the body.) It is a large vein, but it lies very close to the brachial artery. The brachial nerve runs very close to this vein, and in some patients, the nerve may even cross over the vein. If you must use this site to draw and you miss, stop the draw. Do not readjust. A readjustment may result in the needle hitting the nerve.

There are situations in which venipuncture is contraindicated or not necessary, and a finger stick or a heel stick is used to obtain a blood sample. These procedures are not venipunctures because they access capillaries, not veins.

When performing a capillary puncture on an adult, use the middle or ring finger for a finger stick. The little finger is too thin, and the bone is too close to the surface. The index finger and the thumb are likely to be too sensitive or to have thick calluses. It is preferable to use the side of the finger for the stick. The tip of the finger is more sensitive, has fewer capillaries, and can have calluses. Never perform a finger stick on a finger that is cold, cyanotic (blue), scarred, swollen, or has a rash. If you are not sure whether the finger is suitable for a finger stick, use another finger or check with your supervisor. If the finger is thickly callused, choose another finger.

As a new phlebotomist, you will want to seek advice from your colleagues or supervisor before making the decision to collect a capillary specimen instead of a venous specimen, especially with new patients. For established patients, whether in the hospital or an outpatient setting, the lab requisition may state "finger stick specimen," or patients may alert you to collect the specimen from their finger. For infants younger than 12 months, use a heel stick to obtain capillary blood. The veins of infants are too small for a standard venipuncture, and infants do not have sufficient tissue on their fingers for a finger stick. Heel sticks can be used for almost any blood test. The procedure may differ depending on where you work, but if you use the basic techniques outlined below, you can be confident that you are able to perform a heel stick safely.

Select a Site that Minimizes Patient Risk

To begin looking for a suitable vein, it is important to know the acceptable locations on the body to draw blood. The preferred location for venipuncture is the antecubital fossa. (Note: Ante means before, and cubital refers to the elbow joint. Fossa means channel or hollow place.) The antecubital fossa is the area of skin that is between the forearm and the upper arm. It is commonly known as the fold of the elbow, and it can be seen when the patient extends his arm and turns the arm palm up. The antecubital fossa is a good site for venipuncture because there are several large veins there that are close to the surface and easily seen. There are other veins you may use for venipuncture, but these should be last resorts. Use these only when the antecubital veins are unavailable. The other veins you may use for venipuncture are the following:

- Hand veins: Veins of the **dorsal** side of the hand are the next choice after the antecubital fossa. However, these veins are more fragile than the veins in the antecubital fossa, often roll, and are small. Venipuncture of the veins on the dorsal side of the hand is more painful than venipuncture of a vein in the antecubital fossa. Also, because these veins are relatively short and thin, it is difficult to achieve a good angle for a venipuncture, and it is relatively easy to push the needle completely through the vein. When drawing from a hand vein, it is often better to use a butterfly needle. These are easier to guide into smaller veins and may provide more control for the phlebotomist.

- Ankle and foot veins: The veins of the ankle or the foot should be the last choice for a venipuncture. These veins are difficult to access and relatively easy to injure, and venipuncture of these veins is painful. Do not draw from the ankle or foot vein of a diabetic patient. The circulation of the lower extremities can be compromised by common medical problems such as diabetes and peripheral vascular disease. Venipuncture could cause harm through infection, **phlebitis**, or hematoma. Some health care facilities prohibit the use of these veins for venipuncture, or allow them to be used only with a physician's approval.

New or inexperienced phlebotomists should not draw blood from a patient's ankle or foot without first obtaining permission from a nurse or physician. All phlebotomists should take care to know their facility policy on alternative sites for venipuncture before attempting a specimen collection beyond the arm or hand.

Once you have decided which location will be the safest and easiest to use, the next step is to **palpate** the vein. Palpation is a medical term that means touching with the fingers. The purpose of palpating a vein is to determine whether there is any condition that would make the vein unsuitable for a venipuncture. A vein that is suitable for venipuncture should be soft, flexible, and feel spongy or bouncy. Once a vein is felt, palpate for depth, direction, and dimension. Knowing the depth will assist in deciding the angle of insertion. Knowing the direction of the vein will help in ensuring the needle will be in the lumen of the vessel and not pierce through the vein. Knowing the dimension or size of a vein will assist in the choice of the appropriate needle to perform the venipuncture.

There may be times when you cannot visually identify or palpate a vein that seems suitable for a venipuncture. In this case, place the patient's arm below the level of the heart for several minutes. This decreases the return of blood to the heart and allows the veins to fill. A warm compress may be applied to the arm, as well. The heat will dilate the veins, and they will be easier to palpate. However, before applying a warm compress, check to see whether there is a protocol that outlines how the compress should be applied, and check with the patient's nurse to make sure a compress would be safe. A compress that is too hot or improperly applied can be dangerous. Never slap or hit a patient's hand to attempt to make veins more accessible.

There are conditions that indicate you should not draw blood from an area that is normally considered an acceptable site for venipuncture.

Never perform venipuncture from the following:

- Above an IV line in a patient's arm: Intravenous fluids can mix with the blood sample and affect the results.

- In an arm that has a dialysis shunt: The circulation in an arm with a dialysis shunt can be compromised.

- On the same side of the body where the patient had a mastectomy: Lymph nodes are sometimes removed during a mastectomy, diminishing the patient's circulation and ability to fight infection in the area of a venipuncture. If a patient has had a double mastectomy, the physician may perform the draw or determine an arm that is safe for venipuncture.

- Any site that has **edema**: Excess fluid that accumulates in the area may alter test results. It also may be very painful for the patient.

- Any site that is scarred: A draw from a scarred site may make the blood collection difficult and increase pain to the patient.

- Any site that has a **hematoma**: The test results may be altered. It also may cause more pain to the patient, increase the risk of nerve damage by making the hematoma larger, or cause permanent damage to circulation in that limb.

Veins can be large and easily visible but not be a good choice for a venipuncture. Examples of these include the following:

- **Sclerotic** veins: As people age, oftentimes veins become sclerotic. Sclerotic veins are hard, inflexible, and narrow, and they can be difficult to puncture.

- **Tortuous** veins: Tortuous veins are twisted. They do not run in a straight line, and it would be easy to push the needle completely through the wall of these veins.

- **Thrombotic** veins: A vein with a thrombus can feel hard and inflexible and can be tender to the touch.

- Fragile veins: Fragile veins are usually quite thin, and they are not strong. When palpated, they collapse easily and do not refill quickly. Many elderly people have veins that are fragile.

- Phlebitic veins: A vein that is phlebitic will be tender and warm to the touch, and the area around the vein can appear red. Phlebitic veins also can have clots in them.

Performing a venipuncture on a vein that is fragile, sclerotic, or phlebitic will be painful for the patient. The veins will damage easily (fragile veins and be difficult to puncture. The blood supply through the veins also can be poor, so the chances of successfully completing the venipuncture will be slight.

Determine Venipuncture Site Accessibility Based on Patient Age and Condition

Factors such as age or medical or mental condition may alter the patient's ability to understand the medical procedure that you need to perform. It is important to assess the patient to determine whether she has the ability to understand what will happen and can tolerate the phlebotomy procedure.

This assessment does not need to be lengthy or complicated. It should take less than a minute and can be done during the identification of the patient. You may gather some of the information by simply looking and listening.

To determine whether the patient can tolerate the procedure, and to determine whether the patient can understand what will happen during the phlebotomy procedure, follow these steps:

- Make sure the patient can easily and accurately provide her personal information.

- Make sure the patient's speech is clear, coherent, and appropriate.

- Determine whether the patient has any medical conditions or is taking any medications that can increase the risk of bleeding. It is always wise to ask patients whether they take aspirin or coumadin (Warfarin), and if they do, ask when they last took a dose.

- Make sure that the patient has been properly prepared for the venipuncture. Some tests, such as a fasting glucose and measurement of serum cholesterol, require the patient to abstain from eating for at least 8 hr prior to the test.

- Ask the patient if she knows what procedure you will perform.

- Ask the patient if she has ever had blood drawn before.

These questions will take little time to ask. Listen to the answers, and observe the patient to see whether she seems uncertain about who she is, where she is, and what is going to be done. If you have concerns about the patient's ability to understand the phlebotomy procedure, stop and contact your supervisor, a nurse, or a physician.

To ensure the patient can tolerate the phlebotomy procedure, perform the following:

- Ask the patient whether she has had any problems during or after a venipuncture. If the patient says yes, find out what the issue was. Was there excessive pain, significant bruising, prolonged bleeding, chest pain, dizziness, fainting, or nausea?

- Look and listen. Does the patient seem anxious? Is there anything about the patient's body language or tone of voice that indicates fear? If so, ask the patient directly if she is afraid and why.

It is also important not to make assumptions about a patient's veins, no matter what age the patient is, before evaluating the sites and palpating the veins. In cases of pediatric blood draws, evaluate which location and what type of blood collection is appropriate for the age of the child. Infants younger than 12 months who are not walking should have blood collections performed on the heel. Never use a lancet that punctures deeper than 2 mm when performing an infant heel puncture. Do not perform a dermal puncture, or finger stick, on the finger of a child younger than 1 year of age because of the size of the finger, which would increase the risk of injury to the patient. When performing a blood draw on a geriatric patient, it should not be assumed that the patient has difficult-to-access veins. Some geriatric patients may have easily accessible veins. Examine and palpate veins in the antecubital fossa in both arms to determine whether the patient has any veins that would be suitable for blood collection. Some geriatric patients are cold. Warming the area may help in the discovery of a vein. If you find no accessible veins after careful examination of a geriatric patient's arms and hands, you may need to consider a dermal puncture. Evaluate every patient, regardless of age, for the blood collection procedure that will result in accurate test results with the least risk of pain and injury to the patient.

Apply Appropriate Antiseptic Agent Using Aseptic Technique

Once you identify the area and find a vein, the site must be cleansed in order to prevent infection and/or transmission of disease. The standard method for cleaning the skin prior to a venipuncture is to briefly scrub the area with 70% isopropyl alcohol. Phlebotomy technicians almost always use isopropyl alcohol swabs. These are pieces of sterile gauze or paper that are saturated with isopropyl alcohol and come in individual packages. There are many micro-organisms present on the surface of the skin, but intact skin prevents these micro-organisms from entering the body and causing an infection. However, when the surface of the skin is broken during a venipuncture, these micro-organisms can enter the body. **Isopropyl alcohol** can significantly reduce the number of micro-organisms on the skin. Isopropyl alcohol is a germicide: It kills micro-organisms. There are many other germicides (e.g., chlorhexidine, ethyl alcohol, and povidine-iodine). All of the germicides can be used to clean the skin prior to venipuncture. However, isopropyl alcohol dries quickly, does not leave a significant residue, is not highly irritating, does not obscure the venipuncture site (unlike povidone-iodine), and is less drying to the skin than other germicides.

To cleanse the skin, open the alcohol swab package, remove the swab, and scrub the venipuncture site using a concentric circular motion starting from the inside and working out. Clean an area 3 to 4 inches in diameter, and then discard the swab. Allow the area to air-dry. Do not blow, wipe, or fan the site to attempt to speed-drying. These actions may increase micro-organisms in the area. Never reuse the swabs. Reusing an isopropyl alcohol swab could spread micro-organisms from one patient to another.

For most venipunctures, isopropyl alcohol is sufficient. When obtaining blood for certain tests, prepare the venipuncture site differently, and do not use isopropyl alcohol. Two examples when isopropyl alcohol is not the appropriate choice are blood cultures and blood alcohol tests. Physicians order blood cultures to detect the presence of micro-organisms in the blood. Most laboratories specify that site preparation for blood cultures include cleansing with povidone-iodine and isopropyl alcohol. (There are additional cleansing agents available for patients who have iodine sensitivity.) When performing a blood alcohol draw, isopropyl or ethyl alcohol should not be used because it may alter test results. It is important to know the rules and protocols of site preparation that are specific to your facility. These should be a part of your orientation and training when you start a new job. If they are not, ask before attempting to process a patient for these tests. Asking is always preferable to having to call a patient to return for another, unnecessary venipuncture.

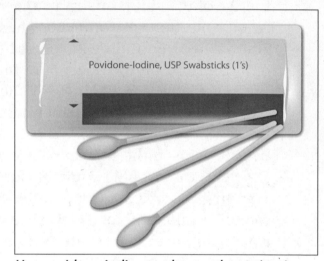

Use povidone-iodine to cleanse the patient's skin before a blood culture.

Verify Patient Compliance with Testing Requirements

Some tests require patient preparation. This may include fasting, taking or not taking medication, having blood collected at a specific time, or a specific body condition. Depending on your work setting, you may have the opportunity to explain these testing requirements to the patient, or you may see patients who arrive with instructions from their doctor's office or other care setting. It is important to know which tests have requirements so you can explain it to or discuss it with the patient. You may occasionally have patients who are not in compliance with the testing requirements present to your phlebotomy station for blood work. If this happens, understand that the patient may be upset, and even angry. Verify the testing requirements, and then talk to the patient in nonmedical terms to ensure that he understands the directions. Ask him to repeat the directions, so you can verify that he understands. Work to schedule another appointment that meets the patient's schedule and allows him to satisfy the pretesting requirements.

Be sure to make the patient comfortable so he may ask any questions, and provide prompt answers to these questions.

Common test preparations include:

- **Fasting**: Some tests require that a patient fast before a test. Often, the patient cannot eat or drink anything other than water for 8 to 12 hr. Unless the patient's condition or procedure expressively prohibits it, encourage the patient to drink water. Some tests allow the patient to drink black coffee or tea. Share this with the patient if applicable.

- Medication: Doctors order some tests to determine the effectiveness of a medication. The patient should take the medication at a predetermined time, or write down what time he takes his medication. Patients will have specific times for the collection of their blood and sometimes urine specimens. Physicians coordinating patient care rely on the accuracy of the timing, so when performing these tests, it is important to collect the specimens at the correct time.

- **Basal state**: This refers to the state, normally first thing in the morning, before the patient eats or exercises, after refraining from both of these activities for the previous 12 hr. This preparation is necessary when the physician wants to establish reference ranges, because exercise and food may affect test results. When educating the patient, be aware that if he works an opposite shift, first thing in the morning may be when the patient is leaving work. In cases such as these, stress the importance of 12 hr of rest, and ask the patient when he can accommodate this in his schedule.

Before performing the test, it is essential to determine whether the patient is in compliance with the requirements for the test. Question the patient using nonmedical terms. For example, ask: "Have you had anything to eat or drink?" Some patients may not understand the term fasting and may respond with yes because many patients know that a positive answer is what the phlebotomist is seeking and will agree to the question even though they do not understand the question. Ensure that the patient provides an exact time that the medication was taken; this will ensure that the blood or urine collection occurs in an appropriate time frame. Some patients may not know what the basal state is, so questions such as, "What time did you wake up?" or "When did you last have anything to eat or drink?" or "Did you exercise today?" help determine whether the patient is in the basal state. It is always important that the patient complies with preparations to help ensure accurate test results.

Summary

Phlebotomy is an invasive procedure because you, as a phlebotomist, disrupt the surface of the patient's skin, and there are complications that can occur. Properly prepare the patient for any blood collection procedure. Preparation begins with a review of the requisition form followed by patient preparation, which involves introduction and patient identification, patient assessment, and education performed in a professional manner. It is essential to obtain the appropriate patient consent before performing any procedure. Before choosing a site for blood collection, assess all sites to help ensure the success of the procedure. Selection of the appropriate site can help decrease patient pain and potential for injury. Appropriate sites may vary from person to person due to underlying conditions, age, injury, or health. Once you choose a site, cleanse using the appropriate antiseptic agent. Before performing a blood draw, it is essential to verify that a patient has met the requirements for the test, such as fasting, taking medication, or resting for the appropriate amount of time.

Drill Questions

1. Which of the following statements is an appropriate introduction to a patient?

   A. "Hello, my name is Courtney. I am a phlebotomy technician and am here to draw your blood."
   B. "Hello, my name is Ms. Johnson. I work at the hospital and am here to test for diabetes."
   C. "Hello. I am a phlebotomist, and I am here to perform a glucose test."
   D. "Hello. I am a phlebotomy technician and need to know if you are fasting."

2. Which of the following is an example of proper patient identification?

   A. Ask the patient where he lives, check the medical record, and check the wristband.
   B. Compare the wristband to the laboratory order sheet, and ask the patient to spell his name.
   C. Ask the patient to state his name and date of birth.
   D. Observe whether the patient answers yes when you call his name.

3. A 19-year-old patient extends her arm and looks away when the phlebotomist enters her hospital room. This is an example of which type of consent?

   A. Expressed
   B. Informed
   C. Implied
   D. Minor

4. A patient has never had his blood drawn before. When explaining the venipuncture procedure, which of the following would be an appropriate statement?

   A. "It will not hurt unless you move."
   B. "It will not hurt. I have done this many times before."
   C. "It may hurt. Tell me if it does."
   D. "It does hurt, but I will perform the draw very quickly."

5. A blood draw must be performed on a 5-month-old infant. Which of the following locations should be the first site choice for the collection?

   A. Scalp
   B. Antecubital area
   C. Finger
   D. Heels

6. Which of the following is the antiseptic of choice for venipuncture?

    A. Isopropyl alcohol
    B. Povidone-iodine
    C. Chlorhexidine
    D. Ethyl alcohol

7. The first step in the patient care process is

    A. assessment.
    B. planning.
    C. information sorting.
    D. follow-up.

8. To inform a patient what preparations should be performed for a test in the basal state, which of the following should the phlebotomist tell the patient?

    A. "The test should be performed right after work."
    B. "The test should be performed first thing in the morning."
    C. "The test requires that a patient records the time she took medication."
    D. "The test requires that the patient records the last time her blood was drawn."

Drill Answers

1. Which of the following statements is an appropriate introduction to a patient?

   A. "Hello, my name is Courtney. I am a phlebotomy technician and am here to draw your blood."
   B. "Hello, my name is Ms. Johnson. I work at the hospital and am here to test for diabetes."
   C. "Hello. I am a phlebotomist, and I am here to perform a glucose test."
   D. "Hello. I am a phlebotomy technician and need to know if you are fasting."

   Phlebotomists must use their names, job title, and what type of test is to be performed. Phlebotomists should not assume what a physician is diagnosing. You may only explain the name of the tests ordered. Verifying the patient's preparation is not part of the introduction.

2. Which of the following is an example of proper patient identification?

   A. Ask the patient where he lives, check the medical record, and check the wristband.
   B. Compare the wristband to the laboratory order sheet, and ask the patient to spell his name.
   C. Ask the patient to state his name and date of birth.
   D. Observe whether the patient answers yes when you call his name.

   Identifying the patient should be an active process, and the patient should be required to provide the proper information. Comparing the laboratory order sheet to the wristband and getting the patient's verbal confirmation is the appropriate patient identification. Although a wristband is one form of ID, the medical record and where a patient lives are not. Verbal information should be compared to documentation for verification. Observing the patient's reaction does not ensure positive identification of the patient.

3. A 19-year-old patient extends her arm and looks away when the phlebotomist enters her hospital room. This is an example of which type of consent?

   A. Expressed
   B. Informed
   C. Implied
   D. Minor

   Implied consent is given when the patient performs an action that indicates that she agrees to the procedure being performed. Expressed consent refers to treatments such as surgery or experimental procedures or medication. Informed consent requires that a patient receives full information about the procedure that is about to be performed. A 19-year-old patient does not need a parent to provide consent.

4. A patient has never had his blood drawn before. When explaining the venipuncture procedure, which of the following would be an appropriate statement?

    A. "It will not hurt unless you move."
    B. "It will not hurt. I have done this many times before."
    C. "It may hurt. Tell me if it does."
    D. "It does hurt, but I will perform the draw very quickly."

The patient must be made aware that the venipuncture may hurt and what actions to take if it does hurt. It is unethical to tell a patient that the procedure will not hurt. The phlebotomist cannot guarantee that the draw will go quickly.

5. A blood draw must be performed on a 5-month-old infant. Which of the following locations should be the first site choice for the collection?

    A. Scalp
    B. Antecubital area
    C. Finger
    D. Heels

The heel is the first choice when performing a blood collection on an infant younger than 12 months old. Scalp veins require special training and are not the first choice. The antecubital region is the first choice in adult patients, not infants. The finger is not used for a patient under 1 year of age due to the risk of damage to the finger.

6. Which of the following is the antiseptic of choice for venipuncture?

    A. Isopropyl alcohol
    B. Povidone-iodine
    C. Chlorhexidine
    D. Ethyl alcohol

Isopropyl alcohol reduces the presence of micro-organisms without leaving a significant residue, significantly drying the skin, or obscuring the site. Povidone-iodine and chlorhexidine are more expensive, leave a residue, and can obstruct the view of a patient's arm. Ethyl alcohol is not the antiseptic of choice for venipuncture.

7. The first step in the patient care process is

   A. assessment.
   B. planning.
   C. treatment.
   D. follow-up.

   Assessment is the process of evaluating and judging. It is the first step in the patient care process – and in phlebotomy – because you assess the patient's needs, fears, abilities, communication skills, medical conditions, and any other factors that can affect the phlebotomy process or the patient's experience. Planning is done after assessment. Phlebotomists do not treat patients. Follow-up is performed after the procedure.

8. To inform a patient what preparations should be performed for a test in the basal state, which of the following should the phlebotomist tell the patient?

   A. "The test should be performed right after work."
   B. "The test should be performed first thing in the morning."
   C. "The test requires that a patient records the time she took medication."
   D. "The test requires that the patient records the last time her blood was drawn."

   Basal state is a 12-hr period of rest and fasting, which is first thing in the morning for most people. After work indicates that the person is not in a state of rest. The time medication was taken is necessary for medication level tests. The patient's last blood draw has no effect on the basal state.

Terms and Definitions

ASAP – As soon as possible

Basal state – State of rest and fasting, normally for at least 12 hr

Dorsal – Back

Edema – A collection of fluid under the skin

Fasting – Not eating or drinking for a period of time, generally at least 8 hr and often 12 hr

Hematoma – A collection of blood underneath the skin, also known as a bruise

Isopropyl alcohol – An antiseptic agent that reduces the presence of micro-organisms on the skin

Medical identification number – Unique number that is established for a patient upon entry to the medical facility

Palpate – To feel with the fingers

Phlebitis – Inflammation of a blood vessel

Requisition form – Form on which tests are ordered; lists pertinent patient information and any special requirements for the test ordered

Sclerotic – Hardened, or veins that are hardened from repeated blood draws

Stat – Immediately, often within 45 min to 1 hr of receipt in the laboratory

Thrombotic – Containing blood clots

Tortuous – Twisted

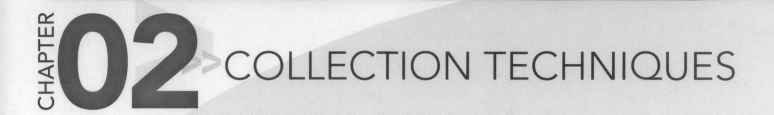

CHAPTER

02 > COLLECTION TECHNIQUES

Learning Objectives

At the end of this chapter, you will be able to:

- *Demonstrate proper insertion and removal techniques for venipuncture.*

- *Perform capillary collection method based on age and condition.*

- *Ensure patient safety through the collection process.*

- *Perform venipuncture steps in correct order (e.g., evacuated tube system, syringe, winged collection set).*

- *Perform capillary (dermal) puncture steps in order.*

- *Recognize common complications from primary collection (e.g., lack of blood flow, hematoma, petechiae, nerve injury).*

- *Identify problematic patient signs and symptoms throughout collection (e.g., syncope, diaphoresis, nausea, seizure).*

- *Follow order of draw when performing venipuncture.*

- *Follow order of draw when performing capillary collection.*

- *Ensure that tube additives are appropriate for testing requirements.*

- *Assemble equipment needed for primary blood collections.*

- *Invert evacuated tubes with additives after collection.*

- *Verify quality of equipment (e.g., sterility, expiration date, manufacturer's defects).*

- *Prepare peripheral blood smears.*

- *Perform blood culture collections.*

- *Assist other health care professionals with blood culture collections.*

- *Collect blood samples for inborn errors of metabolism (e.g., phenylketonuria, galactosemia).*

- *Perform phlebotomy for blood donations.*

- *Calculate volume requirements to avoid causing iatrogenic anemia.*

Overview

Phlebotomists perform venipuncture and capillary collections on patients to collect blood for many tests. These tests help physicians diagnose conditions in their patients, so it is important to take special care to ensure that you perform these collections properly to support accurate test results. Venipuncture refers to blood collection from a vein, usually in the antecubital area, and a capillary collection refers to blood collected from capillaries, usually from the finger or heel. Phlebotomists will use appropriate equipment and devices for all types of blood collection. There is an order of draw that dictates the order in which you draw evacuated tubes. Phlebotomists follow this order of draw to help ensure accurate test results. Observe the patient throughout the entire blood collection procedure in case of complications. When a complication occurs, help to reduce any injury to your patient by providing prompt and appropriate action. Special blood collections address a variety of patient needs and conditions. Peripheral blood smears are made onto glass microscope slides to allow close examination of blood components. The standard method for preparing peripheral blood smears (blood films) is with the wedge smear (push slide) technique. Collect blood cultures using strict antiseptic techniques to prevent contamination of specimens, which could result in an inappropriate antibiotic prescription for the patient. For infants, the standard blood collection process for inborn errors of metabolism involves skin puncture procedures performed on the heel. Some phlebotomists may find work opportunities in blood banks that collect blood for various testing along with collecting blood for transfusions. Phlebotomists may, in consultation with nurses, calculate the impact of frequent venipuncture to ensure that patients, especially infants, are not at risk of developing iatrogenic anemia, which can endanger their health.

Special blood collections are used for a variety of patient needs and conditions. As a phlebotomist, you will find that the practices at different facilities vary. In some locations, you may routinely make blood smears and collect the samples for inborn errors of metabolism. In other facilities, these duties do not fall to the phlebotomy team. In addition, some tasks you will read about in this chapter require additional training and some phlebotomist experience before you will be able to work in these specialty settings. Each work environment will have specific policies, procedures, and practices that guide your work.

Peripheral blood smears are made onto glass microscope slides to allow close examination of blood components. The standard method for preparing peripheral blood smears (blood films) is with the wedge smear (push slide) technique. Blood cultures are collected using aseptic techniques in order to prevent contamination of specimens, which could result in inappropriate antimicrobial therapy. For infants, the standard blood collection process for inborn errors of metabolism involves a heel stick skin puncture procedure. Blood banks collect blood for various blood tests, along with testing and collecting blood for transfusions.

PRIMARY COLLECTIONS

Assemble Equipment Needed for Primary Blood Collections

Depending on your work setting, your equipment setup will vary. In an outpatient setting, such as a doctor's office or lab collection center, you most likely will have a phlebotomy station, where supplies and equipment are kept in a cabinet close to the phlebotomy chair. In the inpatient setting, you may have a phlebotomy tray or cart that you take with you to the inpatient floors. In either setting, you will want to assemble your venipuncture equipment before beginning the procedure and place it in a convenient place next to the patient. Arrange equipment in a location that provides safety for the patient and convenience of use for the phlebotomist.

The equipment used for the evacuated tube system of venipuncture includes the following:

- Gloves: Use a new pair of vinyl or nitrile gloves for each patient venipuncture. The reuse of gloves is prohibited.

- Isopropyl alcohol swabs or pads: Use these to cleanse the skin before inserting the needle. They are to be discarded after each use. The reuse of swabs is prohibited.

- Gauze pads: Use disposable gauze pads to provide pressure to aid in clotting and to cover the venipuncture site. These do not have to be sterile. Reuse of the pads is prohibited.

- Tape or adhesive bandages to keep the clot in place.

- Tourniquet: These are typically made of latex, but other types are available. They can be reused, but if they become soiled or obviously contaminated, they should be discarded.

- Needles: You will use 21- to 23-gauge needles for routine venipuncture. They are sterile and must be disposed of after each use. The 21-gauge needle is the most common size. Never reuse needles.

- Hub or needle holder: This is attached to the needle and used to guide the tubes toward the needle to initiate blood flow into the evacuated tube.

- Evacuated blood collection tubes: Blood collection tubes are glass or plastic tubes that have the capacity to hold blood measured in milliliters (mL). The inside of a blood collection tube is sterile, but the outside is not. The tubes have an opening at one end that is sealed with a rubber stopper. During manufacturing, the air in the tubes is removed, and rubber stoppers are placed over the openings. The tubes then have enough vacuum – negative pressure – that when they are attached to a needle within a vein, blood will flow into the collection tubes. Colored stoppers identify each tube, as does the label on the side of the tube. The color of the stopper indicates which additive is inside. The additives are specific to blood tests, and phlebotomy technicians must know the appropriate tubes to use for each test. Using the incorrect tube can alter the test results.

- Pediatric blood collection tubes: Blood collection tubes used for adults are about 3 inches long and 0.5 to 0.75 inch wide. The vacuum inside adult blood collection tubes is higher than the pressure inside the blood vessels of a child, so an adult collection tube may collapse a child's vein. Pediatric blood collection tubes are identical to adult tubes in color, but they are about half as big and have less vacuum.

- Winged infusion set: A winged infusion set is commonly known as a Butterfly® needle. A winged infusion set consists of a sterile needle, a short length of flexible plastic tubing, and another sterile needle at the other end of the plastic tubing. The second needle is covered with a rubber sheath. Once the first needle has been inserted into the vein, the second needle is used to puncture the rubber collection tube. As the second needle punctures the stopper, the rubber sheath slides back and exposes the lumen on the needle, and blood can flow from the vein into the collection tube.

Demonstrate Proper Insertion and Removal Techniques for Venipuncture

When performing a venipuncture, it is essential to insert and remove the needle correctly to help reduce the risk of injury and pain to the patient. Insert the venipuncture needle bevel up, at a 15° to 30° angle in a swift smooth motion, until a change in resistance is felt. When the needle enters the skin, the phlebotomist will feel resistance, which is the needle penetrating the skin, and must continue insertion. The next feeling is the resistance as the needle penetrates the vessel wall. The insertion should stop when a change is felt in this resistance. This change in feeling indicates that the needle is in the center, or lumen, of the vessel, which is the proper location for the needle during the blood collection. When the venipuncture is complete, remove the needle from the vessel at the same angle as the insertion with the same swift motion.

Perform Capillary Collection Method Based on Patient's Age and Condition

Phlebotomists perform capillary blood draws for tests that require a small amount of blood, or when a patient does not have an accessible vein but a blood collection is essential. Capillary blood draws (called skin punctures or dermal punctures), finger sticks, and heel sticks, are common for many point-of-care (POC) blood tests, including glucose, cholesterol, and **hematocrit**. The patient's age, the ordered tests, and patient's health status may assist in determining whether a venipuncture or capillary blood draw would be the best method of blood collection. For infants, a capillary draw is the preferred method of blood collection because it requires less blood. Infants' veins are small, and numerous venipuncture procedures may result in damage to the vessels. Capillary draws require less blood and therefore reduce the chance of iatrogenic anemia. Some elderly adults may have compromised veins that are difficult to find. In these cases, use a capillary draw to collect the blood for testing. Patients who are underweight also run the risk of iatrogenic anemia. The use of a capillary draw reduces this risk. Even in healthy adults, you may use a capillary blood draw when there is no need for a large volume of blood, when the test is to be performed repeatedly (such as for home glucose testing), or when the test being performed requires capillary blood. In adults, capillary blood draws are performed on the middle or ring finger of the nondominant hand. In infants up to age 1 or before they are walking, capillary blood draws are performed on the infant's heel.

Ensure Patient Safety Throughout the Collection Process

In order to maintain the patient's safety during the phlebotomy procedure, perform a quick, basic assessment of his emotional and physical state in order to determine whether he can tolerate the procedure. Also, be aware of any environmental hazards (e.g., spills or loose sharps). Observe the patient closely to determine whether he is tolerating the procedure.

The majority of patients tolerate venipuncture easily, and most patients report that needle insertion causes only temporary discomfort. However, some people can react strongly to having a needle puncture the skin. In some patients, this reaction may be severe enough to result in the patient experiencing syncope, or fainting. It is essential that the patient begins the blood draw in a safe position. Patients should be sitting in a chair without wheels and preferably with arms. Patients also may be drawn lying down. If the patient reports past experiences of syncope, it is safest to begin the blood draw with the patient lying down. Before the venipuncture begins, inform the patient to tell you if he is feeling any pain, beyond the slight pinch expected with the insertion of the needle. It is advisable to have the patient keep his eyes open so you can monitor them more easily. Always tell the patient that you are going to insert the needle, with a simple statement such as, "you will feel a small poke" or "you will feel a small pinch" immediately before insertion. If the patient states that he is in pain, ask if he wants you to stop the draw. In many cases, the patient will say that he wants the draw to continue. Check with the patient several times during the procedure – talk to the patient – to make sure he is okay. If the patient stops speaking abruptly, ask a question that requires an answer such as "how are you doing?" If he does not respond, this may be a sign of unconsciousness; glance at the patient to determine the patient's status. If the patient is unconscious, the blood collection must be stopped immediately, and first aid measures must be taken. During the blood collection if the patient ever states that he wishes the draw be stopped, the phlebotomist must stop the draw immediately. Statements may be made during the blood collection to inform the patient about the progress of the draw or when the draw is close to completion. After the blood collection is complete, observe the patient for any signs of potential complications, such as syncope, by looking at his face. Look for any extreme skin tone changes, such as being very pale or very red, because these may be signs of a potential complication. Look also for other signs, such as severe sweating. The patient should not be left alone or allowed to leave until the phlebotomist is confident that the patient is experiencing no complications related to the draw.

In the inpatient or hospital setting, there may be times that you need to ask the nurse for assistance. Agitated patients, patients with uncontrollable tremors, or patients with medical equipment that may interfere with a safe phlebotomy procedure can present a challenge to a safe venipuncture process. When in doubt, ask for help. It is always better to ask for help and not need it than to go it alone and experience an unfortunate incident or accidental needlestick.

Perform Venipuncture Steps in Correct Order

- Introduce yourself to the patient.

- Identify the patient using at least two identifiers.

- Have the patient sit or lie down.

- Wash your hands, and put on gloves.

- Assemble equipment.

- Apply the tourniquet.

- Ask the patient to make a fist on the arm that will be drawn.

- Palpate for a vein.

- Choose the most accessible vein.

- Cleanse the venipuncture site.

- Uncap the needle, and inspect the needle for burrs or blunt edges.

- Stabilize the vein with the thumb of the nondominant hand by gently but firmly pulling down on the skin below the vein.

- Alert the patient that she will feel a "pinch."

- Insert the needle at a 15° to 30° angle.

- Insert an evacuated tube, demonstrating the proper order of draw.

- Ensure blood flow into the tube.

- Ask patient to release the fist.

- Remove tourniquet before 1 min.

- Remove each tube, inverting immediately.

- Remove the needle with the same angle of insertion.

- Dispose of the used needle in the sharps container immediately.

- Provide pressure at the site of the draw.

- Check the site to ensure that it is not still bleeding. If the site is still bleeding, continue to provide pressure.

- Apply bandage.

- Label all specimens collected in front of the patient.

- Thank the patient.

- Observe the patient for any complications, such as syncope, bleeding, or seizure.

- Remove gloves.

- Wash hands.

When a patient has fragile or small veins, a winged infusion set may be chosen. The steps for collection are almost the same as for the evacuated tube system with the following exception: After the needle has been inserted, if the needle is in the vein, there will be a flash of blood at the base of the winged infusion set.

When a patient has easy-to-collapse or fragile veins, a syringe may be chosen to perform the blood collection.

The step-by-step process for performing a syringe draw is the following:

- Introduce yourself to the patient.

- Identify the patient.

- Have the patient sit or lie down.

- Wash hands, and don gloves.

- Assemble equipment.

- Pull the plunger in and out of the syringe to ensure a smooth collection.

- Make sure that there is no air in the barrel of the syringe.

- Calculate how much blood is necessary to fill the tubes for the tests required.

- Determine how much blood will be drawn into the syringe.

- Apply the tourniquet.

- Ask the patient to make a fist on the arm that will be drawn.

- Palpate for a vein.

- Choose the most accessible vein.

- Cleanse the venipuncture site.

- Uncap the needle, and inspect the needle for burrs or blunt edges.

- Stabilize the vein with the thumb of the nondominant hand by gently but firmly pulling down on the skin below the vein.

- Alert the patient that she will feel a "pinch."

- Insert the needle at a 15° to 30° angle.

- Pull back slowly on the plunger with the nondominant hand to collect blood.

- Ask patient to release the fist.

- Remove tourniquet before 1 min.

- Collect correct amount of blood into syringe to fill tubes for the tests required.

- Remove the needle with the same angle of insertion.

- Provide pressure at the site of the draw.

- Check the site to see that it is not still bleeding. If the site is still bleeding, continue to provide pressure.

- Apply bandage.

- Use a transfer device to move blood from the syringe into evacuated tubes in the proper order of draw.

- Invert tubes to mix in additives.

- Dispose of transfer device and syringe in sharps container.

- Label all specimens collected in front of the patient.

- Thank the patient.

- Observe the patient for any complications, such as syncope, bleeding, or seizure.

- Remove gloves.

- Wash hands.

Perform Capillary (Dermal) Puncture Steps in Correct Order

When the testing requires only a small amount of blood, or the patient's condition indicates that a venipuncture is not appropriate, the phlebotomist may need to perform a finger or heel stick (dermal puncture). The step-by-step dermal puncture procedure is the following:

- Assemble the equipment: disposable gloves, isopropyl alcohol swabs (or the antiseptic specified by the workplace), adhesive bandage, gauze, lancet, and microtainers.

- Position the patient. The patient should be sitting or lying down. It can be helpful to have the patient place his hand below the level of the heart.

- Wash hands.

- Don gloves.

- Identify the site. Use the middle or ring finger for a finger stick. The little finger is too thin, and the bone is too close to the surface. The index finger and the thumb are likely to be too sensitive or to have thick calluses. It is preferable to use the side of the finger for the stick. The tip of the finger is more sensitive, has fewer capillaries, and can have calluses. Never perform a finger stick on a finger that is cold, cyanotic (blue), scarred, swollen, or has a rash. If you are not sure whether the finger is suitable for a finger stick, use another finger. If the finger is thickly callused, choose another finger.

- Check the warmth of the hand chosen. A warmed site can increase blood flow up to seven times.

- If the patient's fingers are cold and the blood supply is limited, have the patient open and close his hand a few times or rub his hands together vigorously. You also can instruct the patient to place his hand below the level of the heart for 30 seconds.

- Cleanse the site with isopropyl alcohol. Let air dry.

- Puncture the site with the lancet. Make the puncture perpendicular to the fingerprint lines. This will help the blood form into a large drop that is easy to collect. Cuts made parallel to the fingerprint lines cause the blood to flow down the finger, making the blood more difficult to collect.

  - Many facilities provide and encourage the use of auto-lancets, which regulate the skin puncture depth. This is safer for the patients and simpler for the phlebotomist.

- Wipe away the first drop of blood.

- Allow the blood to drip into the collection tube. Cap the tube when it is filled. If the blood flow is slow or stops, you can have the patient drop the hand below the level of the heart, and you can provide pressure to the first joint of the finger with a press-and-release technique, allowing the blood to form large drops. Do not "scoop" the blood to speed collection because this can affect the accuracy of the test results. If you are collecting multiple tubes, you should have a container for the filled but uncapped tubes while you are collecting another tube. Do not take longer than 2 min to fill each tube. Gently invert tubes to mix.

- After capping the tubes, use a gauze pad and put pressure on the area for several minutes. When the bleeding has stopped, put an adhesive bandage over the puncture site if the patient is an adult or responsible child. Children can remove the bandage and swallow it, and adhesive bandages can irritate or tear the skin of infants.

- Label every specimen before leaving the patient's bedside.

- Thank the patient.

- Observe the patient for any complications.

- Remove gloves.

- Wash hands.

When performing a finger stick for other blood tests, including glucose, cholesterol, or hematocrit, follow the manufacturer's instructions specific for each test. The steps will remain the same with the exception of how the blood is collected and the method the blood is put in the cassette or strip used for the test.

A heel stick is used to obtain capillary blood from infants that are not walking or are younger than 12 months. The veins of infants are too small for a standard venipuncture, and infants do not have sufficient tissue on their fingers for a finger stick. Heel sticks can be used for almost any blood test.

The step-by-step procedure for a heel stick is the following:

- Assemble the equipment: Disposable gloves, a heel warming device (optional), isopropyl alcohol swab (or the antiseptic specified by your workplace), a sterile lancet no deeper than 2 mm, blood collection tubes, and a gauze pad.

- Choose the right lancet. Each lancet will puncture the skin to a specified depth, and you must choose the right one. For example, if the child's weight is equal to or less than 1 kg, choose a lancet that punctures the skin to a depth of 0.65 mm. Never use a lancet that goes deeper than 2 mm.

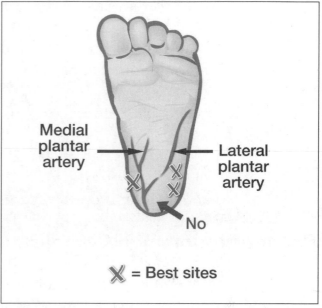

Use only the indicated locations when performing a heel stick.

- Position the patient. If possible, the child should be supine. Check with the patient's nurse or physician to see whether there are restrictions about positioning.

- Apply the heel warmer for 3 to 5 min.

- Wash your hands, and don gloves.

- Select a site. The best sites for a heel stick are the lateral or medial sides of the heel. The skin between the lateral and medial sides should be considered a secondary site. Do not use the back of the heel; there is too little skin/tissue in that area, and a lancet puncture can damage the bone.

- Cleanse the site.

- Place the lancet on the skin, and make the puncture. After the puncture has been made, use your thumb and fingers to gently squeeze the heel. Do not squeeze for a long time or use excessive pressure. Doing so can affect the accuracy of the test results.

- Wipe away the first drop of blood.

- Touch the open tip of the collection tube to the puncture site. The blood should drip into the tube. Allow the blood to passively drip into the tube. Do not "scoop" the blood to speed collection because this can affect the accuracy of the test results.

- If the flow of blood stops, wipe away any surface clots with a gauze pad, and stop squeezing the heel. These actions will remove surface clots that have stopped the blood flow and allow the capillaries to refill.

- When the tubes are filled and capped, use a gauze pad and apply pressure to the site to stop further bleeding.

- Observe patient for any signs of complications.

- Label all tubes before leaving the patient.

- Bandage as appropriate for an infant.

Recognize Common Complications from Primary Collection

One of the more common problems that can occur with venipuncture is that the phlebotomy technician cannot easily see or palpate a suitable vein. You may warm the area to help find a vessel, or lower the arm below the patient's heart. If you cannot find a vessel, ask another phlebotomy technician to try, ask your supervisor for advice, or notify the physician.

Occasionally while performing a venipuncture, the blood flow will stop. You may have advanced the needle too far, causing it to touch the back wall of the vein, or the needle is not deep enough in the vein. The blood collection tubes rarely malfunction, but it is possible for the vacuum in the tube to be insufficient to withdraw blood, or the rubber stopper on the tube may not have been properly punctured. Try another tube. Also, make sure that the tourniquet is no longer on the patient's arm and that the patient is not clenching her fist.

When performing a venipuncture and the blood flow stops or if you perform a venipuncture and no blood is evacuated into the collection tubes, do not repeatedly move the needle in and out, back and forth, or side to side. This is painful for the patient and can cause excessive bleeding and bruising. This also increases the risk of puncturing an artery or a nerve. It is acceptable in these situations to advance the needle slightly. If that does not work, pull it back slightly. But if this does not work, remove the needle.

Some facilities have a policy in place that outlines how many times you may retry phlebotomy. It is generally accepted that a phlebotomist try only twice before asking someone else to collect the sample.

During the venipuncture process, certain complications may occur. Knowing how to identify and address these complications will minimize a patient's pain and risk of permanent injury.

Some complications that may occur during or after a blood draw include the following:

- Nerve damage: If a patient states that she has moderate to severe pain, a sensation of numbness, or a feeling of pins and needles immediately after you insert the needle, it is possible that a nerve has been hit, and you must stop the draw.

- Hematoma: Hematoma is the most common complication associated with phlebotomy. A hematoma is defined as a "localized collection of blood" and occurs through a break in the wall of a blood vessel. Pushing the needle through both walls of the vein can cause a hematoma to form due to the blood that leaks into the surrounding tissue. Hematomas usually disappear in a few days and cause no harm. However, a hematoma can become infected. It also may put pressure on a nearby nerve if it grows too large. If a hematoma starts to appear during the blood collection, stop the draw. Reduce the risk of causing a hematoma by performing venipuncture smoothly and accurately, and by applying the right amount of pressure for the right amount of time after removing the needle.

- Phlebitis: Phlebitis is inflammation of a blood vessel. It usually occurs when the same vein has been accessed repeatedly.

- Thrombus: A thrombus is a blood clot that can occur when insufficient pressure is applied to the venipuncture site.

- Physical reactions: Minor physical reactions, such as diaphoresis (sweating), dizziness, and nausea, can occur during or after a venipuncture, but these are not serious and will usually go away without treatment in a few minutes. Syncope (fainting) is uncommon – it happens in less than 1% of all patients during phlebotomy – but when patients lose consciousness, they can fall and suffer a serious injury. Rarely, a patient who has serious cardiac disease can develop an arrhythmia or a cerebrovascular accident during a syncope episode.

- Petechiae: Petechiae are small red dots that develop on a patient's skin below the tourniquet. They may result due to the routine application of a tourniquet, or in cases where a tourniquet is tied too tightly or left on too long. The chance of petechiae increases with patients who have platelet abnormalities.

- Hemoconcentration: When a tourniquet is tied on too long, the blood flow stagnates in an area, causing hemoconcentration. Hemoconcentration may cause an alteration in test results, especially for ammonia, calcium, coagulation tests, potassium, and protein tests.

- Collection/processing errors: Collection errors are often more common than physical complications, and the consequences of a collection error can be serious or fatal. Examples of collection errors include: misidentification of the patient, improper site selection and preparation, using the wrong tube, incorrect order of the draw, underfilling the tubes, failure to invert the tubes, failing to document the time you obtain or receive a specimen, and mislabeling specimens. The physical complications of venipuncture are visible and distressing to the patient, but it is the collection errors that can cause the most harm.

Identify Problematic Patient Signs and Symptoms Throughout Collection

Phlebotomy technicians also must know what the risks and complications of the phlebotomy procedure are (both to the patient and to the technician), how to prevent them, and what to do if they occur.

As a phlebotomist, you cannot prevent syncope, but it is possible to anticipate it. Ask the patient whether he has ever fainted during a venipuncture. If so, have him lie down, and proceed with the draw cautiously. Also, if the patient seems anxious or if it is his first blood draw, be prepared and on the alert for a syncope episode.

When performing a venipuncture, check for any signs or symptoms that indicate the patient is having difficulty tolerating the procedure. But remember that patients may not, for various reasons, speak up even if they are uncomfortable or in pain. Before the start of the procedure, ask patients to let you know if they are having any problems during or after the venipuncture.

Phlebotomy technicians need to recognize common medical emergencies and know what to do and who to call if one occurs. Typical medical emergencies include the following:

- Syncope: Syncope occurs when there is a sudden lack of blood supply to the brain. It's not unusual for people to faint when blood is being drawn. If a patient faints because of the procedure, it is important to help ensure that he does not fall and suffer injury. However, syncope may be the result of a dangerous medical problem. If someone faints during phlebotomy, never assume that it is simply a reaction to the venipuncture. Keep the patient safe from injury, and immediately call for help. Do not leave the patient alone until he fully recovers. Do not continue to draw blood on a patient who is unconscious.

- Seizure: If a patient begins to have a seizure during blood collection, stop the draw immediately. Stay with the patient, and take steps to help prevent injury to the patient. Call for help. Do not attempt to restrain the patient; this could result in injury to the patient and the phlebotomist alike. Sometimes for several minutes after a seizure, a patient still requires time to fully recover. Do not leave the patient alone.

- Shock: Common symptoms of shock are cold, clammy, and pale skin, rapid pulse, an increase in shallow breathing, and staring eyes in an expressionless face. When you suspect shock, call for help. Ensure that the patient has an open airway. If the patient is lying down, lower the head below the body. Keep the patient warm until help arrives.

- Nausea: A patient may state that he is feeling nauseated, or sick to his stomach. The patient may not say anything but may demonstrate symptoms similar to syncope. If a patient experiences nausea before a draw, wait to perform the blood collection until the patient states that he no longer feels nauseated. If a patient states that he is nauseated during the draw, stop the draw and provide a basin, trash can, or other container in case the patient vomits. Do not resume the draw until nausea is gone. If the patient states that he is nauseated after the draw, provide a basin, trash can, or other container. Do not leave a patient who complains of nausea alone. A cold compress on the patient's head or the back of the neck may help the patient feel better. Never encourage a patient not to vomit, to "hold it in," or to swallow the vomit because it may cause choking. If the patient vomits, provide a wet cloth for the patient to clean off his month. You also may provide a glass of water but only if the patient is not a choking risk or on a fluid restriction. Inform the nurse that the patient has vomited and what actions you took to address it.

- Diaphoresis: Diaphoresis, also known as excessive sweating, may be a sign of nausea, vomiting, syncope, or that a patient is experiencing a panic attack. The sweating itself is not a condition, but it may indicate other underlying difficulties. Do not leave the patient alone until he stops sweating. Provide a disposable cloth for the patient to wipe his face. Observe the patient for other signs, and contact the nurse or physician accordingly.

Follow Order of Draw When Performing Venipuncture

The order of draw is important because the use of a double-sided needle results in additive carryover from one evacuated tube to another during a blood draw. This additive carryover can cause test results to be adversely altered. To ensure the most accurate test results, it is essential to always draw tubes in the correct order of draw. The order of draw for the syringe is the same as the order of draw for venipuncture.

The Clinical and Laboratory Standards Institute's order of draw for venipuncture is as follows:

- Blood culture bottles, or light yellow tube stopper: Blood culture bottles come in sets of aerobic and anaerobic. The light yellow stopper tube contains the additive SPS.

- Light blue: The light blue stopper tube contains the additive sodium citrate.

- Serum tubes: Tube stopper may be red, gold, "speckled" red and gray, or red and black. Serum tubes contain no additive, but may contain a clot activator.

- Green: Green stopper tubes contain the additive heparin.

- Lavender or purple: Lavender, pink, or pearl stopper tubes contains the additive **EDTA.**

- Gray: Gray stopper tubes contain the additives sodium fluoride and potassium oxalate.

Some facilities may routinely order special testing that requires additional (different additive) tubes to be drawn. These would most likely be sequenced after the lavender top tube. In addition, depending on the venipuncture method used, extra care may be required when drawing blue top tubes for coagulation testing. Be sure to check for the standard procedures at your facility so you can be prepared for any phlebotomy request.

Follow Order of Draw When Performing Capillary Collection

The order of draw is equally as important for dermal puncture collections into microtainers. The order of draw for a dermal puncture varies from the order of draw for venipuncture.

The CLSI order of draw for capillary collection is as follows:

- Blood gas collections: Purple, lavender, pink, or pearl cap tubes contain the additive EDTA.

- Green: Green cap tubes contain the additive heparin.

- Any other additive specimens.

- Serum: Red or gold cap tubes contain no additive or clot activator.

Ensure that Tube Additives are Appropriate for Testing Requirements

To ensure accurate test results, the proper additive tube must be chosen to match the blood test that is being performed. Some evacuated tubes contain no additive, and they are used for tests that require that the blood be allowed to clot before being centrifuged and require serum. These tubes are used for draws that require serum and are used for chemistry tests. Other tubes contain anticoagulants that prevent the blood from clotting and are used for tests that require plasma. The anticoagulant that is chosen depends upon the function of the additive on the blood.

Some of the widely used anticoagulants are the following:

- Sodium citrate: Found in the light blue tubes and used for clotting tests because it performs the best at preserving the coagulation factors.

- EDTA: Found in the lavender or pink tubes and used for most hematology tests because it helps preserve the shape of cells and reduces platelet clumping.

- Heparin: Found in green tubes and used for most chemistry tests because it prevents blood clots from causing falsely elevated results, especially in potassium tests.

- Potassium oxalate: Found in grey tubes and used for testing sugar levels because it helps to preserve glucose along with sodium fluoride.

Uses of an improper tube for a blood test can adversely alter the test results.

Invert Evacuated Tubes with Additives after Collection

After filling the tubes with blood, gently invert them to mix the additive with the blood to help ensure accurate blood results and proper clotting. Inverting of tubes should occur as soon as possible after filling to help prevent clotting in tubes and mixing the blood with the anticoagulant. Inverting the tube means holding the tube in your hand and then turning your wrist so that the bottom of the tube points up, and then reversing the movement. An inversion is one complete turn of the wrist. Point the bottom of the tube up and then down. Avoid vigorous shaking, overinverting, or inverting roughly. A gentle inversion will help avoid hemolyzing the blood sample and contributes to accurate test results. The number of inversions will vary depending on the color of the tube.

In general, follow these guidelines:

- Light yellow SPS top tubes: 8 to 10 inversions

- Light blue top tubes: 3 to 4 inversions

- Serum separator tubes (SST, red tops) and serum tubes (red tops without the separating gel): 5 inversions

- Green top tubes: 8 to 10 inversions

- Lavender top tubes: 8 to 10 inversions

- Gray top tubes: 8 to 10 inversions

Verify Quality of Equipment (e.g., Sterility, Expiration Date, Manufacturer's Defects)

Check all blood drawing equipment to determine that it meets quality control standards to support safe blood collection for the patient and phlebotomist alike. Check the equipment that is in the phlebotomy tray or in storage on a routine basis for expiration dates and any corruption of the equipment, such as missing labels, defects, cracks, or breaks. Perform these checks with every blood draw.

Examine needles for:

- Expiration date, and do not use if expired.

- Labels/seals, and if broken, do not use because they may no longer be sterile.

- Intact bevel, and if there are burrs or other flaws, do not use the needle.

- Safety device, and do not use if safety device is missing or broken.

Needles must be used only once, and safety devices must always be deployed. Dispose of any needle that is expired, that has a broken label, a damaged bevel, or doesn't have a safety device into a sharps container.

Evacuated tubes have an expiration date. Do not use beyond that date. Additives in expired tubes may not work correctly and may alter test results. Also, the vacuum in an expired tube may be insufficient to guarantee a complete blood collection. Do not use tubes missing a label. Inspect all tubes for cracks or breaks in the tube or stopper. Do not use, and discard any tubes that are expired, cracked, without a label, or have any other defects.

Check your adapter. Some are single-use, and you will discard after using once. Others are multiple-use. Before use, inspect for any manufacturer's defects, cracks, or breaks. Dispose of any adapters that are cracked, broken, or contaminated.

SPECIAL COLLECTIONS

Prepare Peripheral Blood Smears

A **blood smear** is a thin film of blood that is spread onto a glass slide. Blood smears are used to microscopically examine the blood. Either venous blood in a tube or capillary blood collected by dermal puncture may be used. Blood smears also can be prepared by applying blood directly from a finger onto the slide. Well-made **peripheral blood smears** are important for obtaining accurate health information for patients.

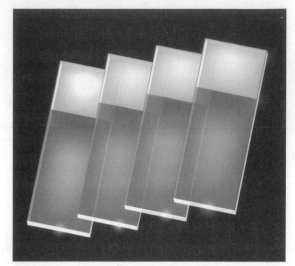

Use glass slides for blood smears.

Phlebotomists may assist laboratory personnel by preparing blood smears. If a smear is needed to confirm abnormal findings, it is best when made fresh and must be prepared within 1 hr of collection in an EDTA tube. Therefore, blood smears are sometimes made at outpatient facilities such as physicians' offices. Prepare blood smears on glass slides using a wedge method. This is defined as the touching of two slides at an angle, which forms a wedge shape. Most large laboratories use an automated slide-maker, which creates a perfect thin smear with the push of a button. These are available in fixed and portable versions and produce consistent, high-quality smears that stain well and support high-quality results. Both techniques – automated and by hand – produce thin smears from fresh, anticoagulated drops of blood.

The steps to perform a manual slide smear are as follows:

- Assemble the equipment needed for dermal puncture, or obtain a tube of uncoagulated blood (usually containing EDTA).

- Make sure you have at least two clean glass microscope slides.

- If performing a dermal puncture:

  - Wipe away the first drop of blood with a piece of gauze.

  - Squeeze the first finger joint to obtain a free-flowing drop of blood.

  - Allow this drop of blood to fall onto the glass slide toward one end.

- If preparing smears using tubes of blood, make sure to check the specimen for proper labeling.

- Use a safety device to access the blood. If no safety device is available, carefully uncap the specimen tube behind a safety shield and use a disposable pipette or plastic dropper to remove some of the blood. You may also use applicator sticks or a capillary tube to place the drop on the slide.

- Place the slide on a flat work surface, and apply a drop of blood onto the slide about ½ inch from the frosted end.

- Discard the applicator stick or capillary tube into a sharps container.

- Pick up the spreader slide with your dominant hand, holding it at a 30° to 35° angle.

- Place the edge of the spreader slide on the smear slide close to the unfrosted end.

- Pull or "back up" the spreader slide toward the frosted end until the spreader slide touches the blood drop. (Action of the capillaries will spread the droplet along the edge of the spreader slide.)

- Let the blood drop spread almost to the edges of the spreader slide.

- Push the spreader slide toward the clear end of the slide (with one light, smooth, fluid motion) until you come off the end – maintain the 30° to 35° angle.

- Label with the patient information using a permanent marker, or aliquot label.

- Allow the smear to air dry before staining.

Note: Most of the drop should be spread out onto the glass slide. It will be thicker at the drop and thinner at the opposite end. If properly made, there will be a critical area used for performing the differential, and a "tail" with a feathered edge that is slightly rounded. Blood smears should not touch the edges of the glass slide. They should appear smooth, without irregularities, streaks, or holes.

Reminder: Make sure the frosted side is facing upward when you use slides that have a frosted end. Do not place the drop of blood directly on the frosted end – it is used to write the patient information or to affix an aliquot label.

Perform Blood Culture Collection

A **blood culture** is a laboratory test used to check for bacteria or other micro-organisms in a blood sample. Physicians order this test to help diagnose conditions in patients who have a fever of unknown origin.

Phlebotomists working in hospitals – especially those with a busy emergency department – may see a lot of blood culture orders. The blood sample is sent to a laboratory where it is placed into a special dish and observed to see whether micro-organisms grow (this is the actual "culture"). If this occurs, further tests will be done to identify the specific micro-organisms present.

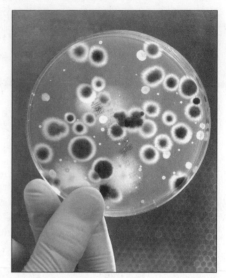

Blood cultures check for bacteria and other micro-organisms.

When performing a blood culture, follow these steps:

- Properly identify the patient.

- Wash hands, and don gloves.

- Assemble supplies, including a winged infusion set or syringe needle, adapter, and blood culture collection bottles.

- Mark blood collection bottles with the level of blood required.

- Remove protective cap, and cleanse the top of the blood collection bottles.

- Apply tourniquet.

- Palpate to find accessible blood vessel, then remove tourniquet while you prepare the skin.

- Clean the intended area of venipuncture for 60 seconds first with alcohol or chlorhexadine gluconate. Apply light friction using an outward spiral technique from the site by placing the swab on the venipuncture site and moving outward, using concentric circles to a diameter of 2 to 2.5 inches.

- Allow the area to dry completely.

- Cleanse the area again, using the outward spiral, taking care to cover the entire 2- to 2.5-inch area, this time using povidone-iodine.

- Do not touch this area after it has been cleansed, and allow it to dry completely.

- Reapply the tourniquet after you are sure the area has dried.

- Ask the patient to clench her hand into a fist.

- Stretch the skin downward below the collection site, using the thumb of your nondominant hand to anchor the vein in place.

- Quickly insert the needle into the vein at a 15° to 30° angle with the bevel facing up. Pop the blood culture bottle onto the double-pointed needle. (If the blood culture set includes aerobic and anaerobic, the aerobic is collected first.)

- Have the patient unclench her fist as blood enters the tube or bottle.

- As each tube is removed from the needle holder, gently invert to properly mix the specimen.

- Remove the tourniquet before 1 min.

- Monitor the patient's condition.

- Make sure not to disturb the needle's position as tubes fill.

- Quickly remove the needle using the same angle as insertion.

- Apply gauze, using pressure, to the puncture site.

- Activate the safety device so that the needle is immediately covered.

- Dispose of the entire needle assembly into a sharps container.

- Make sure that the vein is not leaking by conducting a two-point check, observing the site for up to 10 seconds after releasing pressure and removing the gauze. If visible bleeding occurs (or if the surrounding tissue rises), keep applying pressure until bleeding stops.

- Apply a bandage or tape clean gauze over the puncture site.

- Label all blood collection bottles and tubes, if any, before leaving the patient.

- Check the patient's status again.

- Leave the room or dismiss the patient.

Assist Other Health Care Professionals with Blood Culture Collections

At times, other health care professionals may need to assist with blood culture collections. This may involve notifying the proper laboratory person when the culture is to be done, assembling all needed materials, and explaining procedures to patients. When assisting with blood cultures, you may perform the following actions:

- Obtaining and labeling proper tubes or bottles

- Carefully washing hands before the procedure

- Observing standard precautions by putting on gloves as well as providing gloves for the person you are assisting

- Placing a protective pad under the patient's arm

- Preparing the patient's skin, usually with at least two antiseptic wipes

- Assisting in the actual drawing of blood

- Helping to place folded gauze pads tightly over the venipuncture site, and securing them firmly with tape

- Checking the patient a few minutes later to make sure bleeding has stopped

- Assisting with the proper disposal of all supplies

- Documenting that the procedure was done, and who performed it

- Immediately taking the specimens to the laboratory – inappropriate growth may occur if the specimens are not handled correctly

Collect Blood Samples for Inborn Errors of Metabolism (e.g., PKU, Galactosemia)

In the United States, newborns must be tested for various disorders, including cystic fibrosis, hypothyroidism, **phenylketonuria** (PKU), and **galactosemia**. These genetic diseases are explained briefly as follows:

- Cystic fibrosis – mucous secretions that accumulate in various organs

- Hypothyroidism – decreased thyroid function

- PKU – a buildup of phenylketone caused by decreased metabolism of phenylalanine

- Galactosemia – the inability to break down galactose, a milk sugar

Other genetic disorders, such as deficiency of the enzyme that breaks down biotin (*biotinidase deficiency*) and abnormal hemoglobin structure (*sickle cell disease*), also may be tested for in various states. Other testing may be done for infectious diseases, such as human immunodeficiency virus (HIV) and toxoplasma. Testing is done after each baby is 24 hr old. State-required blood tests are collected onto special forms. These include absorbent areas called filter paper for the specimens. Fill out the forms completely in ink with all required information, and check the forms for expiration dates because the substances within the absorbent areas may expire.

To perform a heel stick, or **dermal puncture**, on an infant's heel, you must follow the procedures listed on the state form(s). A common order of steps that are followed for collecting these samples is as follows:

- Properly identify the infant.

- Check to ensure that paperwork is filled out completely.

- Wash hands, and don gloves.

- Check temperature of the infant's heel, and warm if necessary.

- Cleanse the infant's heel, and allow the skin to dry.

- Puncture the heel with a lancet no deeper than 2 mm.

- Wipe off the first drop of blood.

- Allow a large blood droplet to form.

- Touch the filter paper to the drop of blood to soak through completely in each circle. The circles must be totally saturated – this is evident by viewing the paper from both sides. Note: Blood is applied to only one side of the form.

- Do not use capillary tubes because they often make the filter paper rough and cause overabsorption.

- Air dry the blood spots thoroughly for 3 hr at room temperature. (They must be kept away from direct sunlight and heat.)

- Wet filter papers should not come into contact with each other because they are sticky and will adhere to other forms.

Note: These specimens may be unusable and rejected if any of the following occurs:

- A circle is oversaturated.

- All circles are not completely filled.

- An expired form is used.

- The form is not received within 14 days of collection.

- The specimen is contaminated with a foreign substance.

- The specimen is not allowed to dry thoroughly.

State collection forms, once thoroughly dried, are mailed to appropriate state laboratories for testing.

Perform Phlebotomy for Blood Donations

Phlebotomists with experience and additional training may find work opportunities in a **blood bank** or regional blood center. These facilities are responsible for collection, processing, and storing blood for transfusions and other purposes. The blood bank department in a hospital is usually part of the laboratory, and serves as the screening and release point for donor units and other blood products that patients may need. Blood bank departments work closely with regional blood centers that provide blood and blood products to hospitals for dispensing to patients upon physician request. In larger facilities, the hospital blood bank may draw donor units, but increasingly, these duties reside in the regional blood centers that serve a community or region.

Blood banks also may perform **therapeutic phlebotomy**, which is the intentional removal of blood to lower red blood cell (polycythemia vera: high red blood cell count) or iron levels (hemochromatosis: exceedingly high iron levels). How facilities choose to assign this procedure will vary from organization to organization. Some facilities will refer patients to the regional blood center, and others will assign laboratory professionals – often medical technologists – to perform the procedure. Still other others will assign therapeutic phlebotomy to nursing.

In blood collection for blood bank specimens, it is critical to avoid misidentification of the patient to prevent fatal transfusion errors. The process follows these steps:

- Properly identify the patient as you would with any blood draw, using at least two patient identifiers.

- Perform the venipuncture procedure, and collect the appropriate tubes. This is often a plain red-top tube and an EDTA tube.

- Label the specimens with special blood bank labels in the presence of the patient. (Follow the procedure required by your laboratory.)

- Recheck information by comparing the labels on the tubes with the patient armband or specific blood bank identification band.

- Carry out post-venipuncture patient care.

- Deliver the specimens and blood bank requisition to the blood bank or your facility's transfusion service as soon as possible.

Collecting Donor Blood

Donated blood can be processed into various blood products, including red blood cells, plasma, and platelets. **Apheresis** techniques allow the removal of one or more of these blood products during blood collection via special equipment. *Plasmaphoresis* is the removal of blood plasma from whole blood.

For each donor, a mini-physical examination is given, including taking of the donor's temperature, pulse, and blood pressure. A health history is taken, including questions about sexual activity, recent out-of-country travel, and use of medications.

Autologous Blood Donation

The term **autologous** refers to "self," and today, many individuals donate blood for their own future use. This type of donation has become popular due to increased concern of the transmission of HIV/AIDS and other blood-borne pathogens. If the patient is donating blood before a surgical procedure, he must have a written order from a health care provider and must be in good health so the donation does not stress his body before surgery. The hemoglobin must be at least 11 grams/dL, and the surgical procedure must be scheduled for more than 72 hr after the autologous blood donation. Autologous blood is collected in the same manner as donor blood collection but is labeled strictly for the donor's use and may not be crossed over into the general blood supply.

Calculate Volume Requirements to Avoid Causing Iatrogenic Anemia

Iatrogenic anemia is caused by blood loss due to repeated venipunctures. Geriatric, underweight, and pediatric patients are most susceptible to phlebotomy-induced anemia. In most health care organizations, the role of monitoring patient status to prevent conditions like anemia will be a nursing responsibility. However, it is a good idea for phlebotomists to understand the implications of drawing too much blood in a short period of time, and to be willing to communicate any concerns with the appropriate health care professional. If you have a venipuncture request that seems excessive for a patient, always check with the nurse to ensure that the patient will not be put at risk.

For infants, no more than 10% of blood volume should be drawn in a short period of time. For adults, more than 100 mL may result in a decrease in hemoglobin or hematocrit.

To calculate infant blood volume, perform this calculation:

- Convert the infant's weight from pounds to kilograms. Divide pounds by 2.2 (for example, 6.2 lbs / 2.2 = 2.82 kg).

- Multiply the number of kilograms by 100 (for example, 2.82 x 100 = 282 mL).

- Convert blood volume in mL to liters (for example, 282 mL / 1,000 = 0.28 L).

The actual amount of blood collected in each tube must be documented so that, over time, calculation of total amount of blood removed can be ascertained.

The minimum required amount of blood, therefore, must always be drawn in order to avoid causing iatrogenic anemia, which can lead to shortness of breath, fatigue, and the need for blood transfusions.

As a phlebotomist, you will want to communicate regularly with your supervisor or the laboratory manager to provide the best care for all patients. Discuss any concerns that you may have about physician ordering patterns, or the timing of a patient's draw requests with your supervisor (or the laboratory supervisor).

Summary

Blood smears are used to microscopically examine blood. The results are used with other tests to diagnose many different disorders. Blood smears are prepared on glass slides. Blood cultures test for bacteria or other micro-organisms. Other health care professionals may assist with obtaining blood cultures. Newborns are screened for a variety of disorders 24 hr after birth. State-required blood tests are collected onto special paper forms, using heel punctures. Blood banks collect blood for transfusions and other purposes. Ensuring a safe blood supply is critical. Care must be taken to avoid too many venipunctures from a single patient in order to avoid iatrogenic anemia.

Drill Questions

1. Which of the following is the appropriate angle to hold the slide when preparing a peripheral blood smear?

    A. 20° to 25°
    B. 30° to 35°
    C. 40° to 45°
    D. 45° to 50°

2. What is a blood culture primarily used to check for?

    A. Blood typing
    B. Pregnancy
    C. Bacteria
    D. Platelets

3. For which of the following is testing of newborns required in all states of the United States?

    A. Anti-A titers
    B. Phenylketonuria
    C. Human immunodeficiency virus
    D. Sickle cell disease

4. When state-required testing of an infant's capillary blood is done, which of the following must occur?

    A. The blood is dropped onto both sides of the filter paper.
    B. Capillary tubes are used along with the filter paper.
    C. The blood spots are dried in direct sunlight.
    D. The circles on the filter paper must be totally saturated.

5. For which condition is therapeutic phlebotomy commonly used?

    A. Iatrogenic anemia
    B. Hemophilia
    C. Iron deficiency
    D. Polycythemia vera

6. A patient can donate blood if he or she

   A. is 13 years old, with parent permission.
   B. weighs less than 110 pounds.
   C. donated blood 9 weeks ago.
   D. is negative for AIDS but positive for HIV.

7. Which term is used to describe a blood donation from a patient for later use in his or her own surgical procedures?

   A. Transfused
   B. Autologous
   C. Autotransplantation
   D. Autoimmunity

8. In a hospitalized patient whose blood may be drawn every day or every few hours, what type of anemia is commonly seen?

   A. Hemolytic
   B. Sickle cell
   C. Iatrogenic
   D. Pernicious

Drill Answers

1. Which of the following is the appropriate angle to hold the slide when preparing a peripheral blood smear?

    A. 20° to 25°
    B. 30° to 35°
    C. 40° to 45°
    D. 45° to 50°

    A 30° to 35° angle is appropriate when preparing a peripheral blood slide.

2. What is a blood culture primarily used to check for?

    A. Blood typing
    B. Pregnancy
    C. Bacteria
    D. Platelets

    A blood culture is primarily used to check for the presence of bacteria or other micro-organisms in the blood. It is not useful for blood typing, detecting pregnancy, or checking for platelet antibodies.

3. For which of the following is testing of newborns required in all states of the United States?

    A. Anti-A titers
    B. Phenylketonuria
    C. Human immunodeficiency virus
    D. Sickle cell disease

    All of the states require newborn testing for phenylketonuria. Only certain states require testing for human immunodeficiency virus and sickle cell disease. Anti-A titers testing is done when adults donate blood.

4. When state-required testing of an infant's capillary blood is done, which of the following must occur?

    A. The blood is dropped onto both sides of the filter paper.
    B. Capillary tubes are used along with the filter paper.
    C. The blood spots are dried in direct sunlight.
    D. The circles on the filter paper must be totally saturated.

The circles on the filter paper must be totally saturated when state-required testing of an infant's capillary blood is done. The blood must be applied to only one side of the filter paper, without using capillary tubes, and should be kept away from direct sunlight as it dries.

5. For which condition is therapeutic phlebotomy commonly used?

    A. Iatrogenic anemia
    B. Hemophilia
    C. Iron deficiency
    D. Polycythemia vera

Therapeutic phlebotomy is commonly used for polycythemia vera. Latrogenic anemia may be caused by overuse of phlebotomy, wherein too much blood volume is collected over time. Therapeutic phlebotomy is not indicated for hemophilia and would actually be harmful for iron deficiency.

6. A patient can donate blood if he or she

    A. is 13 years old, with parent permission.
    B. weighs less than 110 pounds.
    C. donated blood 9 weeks ago.
    D. is negative for AIDS but positive for HIV.

A healthy adult (meaning age 18 and up), weighing at least 110 pounds, without HIV/AIDS or any other transmissible disease, can donate blood after 8 weeks.

7. Which term is used to describe a blood donation from a patient for later use in his or her own surgical procedures?

    A. Transfused
    B. Autologous
    C. Autotransplantation
    D. Autoimmunity

An autologous blood donation is one that a patient donates for his or her own later use, including in surgical procedures. The term "transfused" simply means intravenous transfer of blood. "Autotransplantation" means the transplantation of organs, tissue, or proteins from one part of a patient's body to another. "Autoimmunity" is the failure of an organism to recognize its own constituent parts as "self," allowing an immune response against its own cells and tissues.

8. In a hospitalized patient whose blood may be drawn every day or every few hours, what type of anemia is commonly seen?

    A. Hemolytic
    B. Sickle cell
    C. Iatrogenic
    D. Pernicious

Iatrogenic anemia is caused by blood loss due to repeated venipunctures, which is common in hospitalized patients whose blood is drawn regularly. Hemolytic anemia, sickle cell anemia, and pernicious anemia are not caused by repeated venipunctures.

Terms and Definitions

Apheresis – The removal of whole blood from a patient or donor; the components of whole blood are separated mechanically, one of the separated portions is withdrawn, and the remaining components are transfused back into the patient or donor

Autologous – "Self;" in blood transfusion and transplantation, it means that the donor and recipient are the same person

Blood bank – A place where blood is collected from donors, typed, separated into components, stored, and prepared for transfusion to recipients; a blood bank may be a separate free-standing facility, or part of a larger laboratory in a hospital

Blood culture – A laboratory test used to check for bacteria or other micro-organisms in a blood sample

Blood smear – A blood test performed on slides that gives information about the number and shape of blood cells

Dermal puncture – Also known as a skin puncture; a procedure in which a finger or heel is lanced to obtain a small quantity of blood for testing; also called a capillary draw

EDTA – Ethylenediaminetetraacetic acid; used as an anticoagulant to keep blood specimens from clotting

Galactosemia – An inherited disorder in which the body is unable to use (metabolize) the simple sugar *galactose*, causing the affected patient to be unable to tolerate any form of milk, as well as other foods containing galactose

Hematocrit – The proportion of the blood that consists of packaged red blood cells, expressed as a percentage by volume; the *hematocrit* test measures the percentage of hematocrit in the blood

Iatrogenic anemia – A type of anemia that results from multiple phlebotomies; it is especially common in geriatric, pediatric, or underweight patients

Peripheral blood smears – Also called blood films; they consist of a thin layer of blood smeared on a microscope slide and then stained to allow microscopic examination

Phenylketonuria – Abbreviated as PKU; a metabolic genetic disorder characterized by a deficiency in the hepatic enzyme phenylalanine hydroxylase; the form known as *classic PKU* causes permanent intellectual disability, seizures, delayed development, behavioral problems, psychiatric disorders, a "mousy" body odor, lightening of skin and hair, and eczema

Therapeutic phlebotomy – A form of phlebotomy prescribed as treatment for patients with polycythemia vera (high red blood cell count) or hemochromatosis (high iron count)

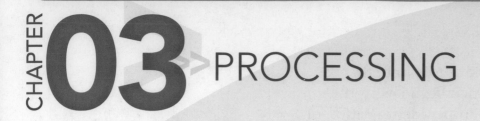

CHAPTER 03 PROCESSING

Learning Objectives

At the end of this chapter, you will be able to:

- *Label all specimens.*

- *Perform quality control for CLIA-waived procedures.*

- *Transport specimens based on handling requirements (e.g., temperature, light, time).*

- *Explain nonblood specimen collection procedures to patients (e.g., stool, urine, semen, sputum).*

- *Handle patient-collected nonblood specimens.*

- *Avoid preanalytical errors when collecting blood specimens (e.g., QNS, hemolysis).*

- *Adhere to chain of custody guidelines when required (e.g., forensic studies, blood alcohol, drug screen).*

- *Prepare samples for transportation to a reference (outside) laboratory.*

- *Coordinate communication between nonlaboratory personnel for processing and collection.*

- *Use technology to input and retrieve specimen data.*

- *Report critical values for point-of-care testing.*

- *Distribute laboratory results to ordering providers.*

Overview

It is important for phlebotomists to understand the processing procedures required for many different tests. For each test to be accurate, quality control is essential. Common nonblood specimens include urine, stool, semen, and sputum.

Errors in various types of collection may go unnoticed, causing inaccurate results and possible rejection, requiring re-collection of specimens. Chain-of-custody guidelines help maintain control of and accountability for specimens used for forensic studies, blood alcohol testing, and drug screening. Samples must sometimes be sent to reference laboratories, and proper handling is essential to ensure accurate test results.

Label All Specimens

Phlebotomists play an important role in high-quality laboratory testing, which begins with the identification of the patient. Proper identification of the patient prior to drawing blood, as you already know, is the first step, but you must also take care to properly label each specimen before leaving the patient room or the drawing station. Many hospitals or laboratories require phlebotomists to initial and mark the date and time of the draw on the label for each specimen. This enables the lab to track the specimen's path if there is ever a question. Be sure to learn the requirements at your facility for accurately documenting each specimen and properly identifying the patient whose blood or body fluid you are submitting for testing.

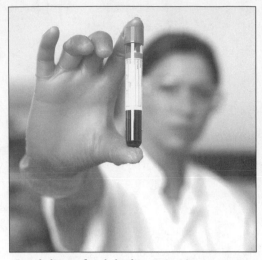

Guidelines for labeling specimens vary by facility.

Perform Quality Control for CLIA-Waived Procedures

The Clinical Laboratory Improvement Act (CLIA) establishes guidelines for certain tests that may be performed in both a patient's home and medical facilities, called CLIA-waived tests. CLIA-waived tests require a minimum of judgment and interpretation and present much less risk to patients because they involve small amounts of blood or other easily obtained specimens, such as urine. These tests include blood glucose by glucose monitoring devices, fecal occult blood, spun microhematocrit, urine chemical screening, and visual color comparison urine tests used for pregnancy. There are many kit tests and will be many more in the future that will be CLIA-waived. Tests also include kit screening tests for point-of-care chemical analyzers, such as cholesterol and drug screens.

Laboratories that perform waived tests will apply for a Certificate of Waiver to achieve CLIA approval. Clinical laboratory professionals oversee this testing at inpatient facilities, ensuring test quality, regulatory compliance, method validation, accuracy, and appropriate test procedures. They also oversee training and technical support. Waived tests, though simple, can still cause serious patient consequences if done incorrectly.

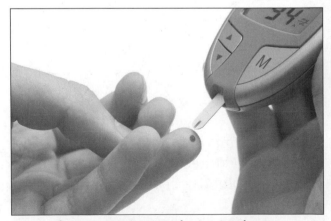

Use a glucose monitoring device, such as a glucometer, to perform a blood glucose test.

Quality control for CLIA-waved procedures includes:

- Confirming written test orders

- Establishing procedures for patient identification

- Giving patients pretest instructions and following up to verify that the patients follow them

- Collecting specimens according to package insert instructions

- Labeling specimens appropriately

- Avoiding use of expired **reagents** or test kits

- Performing quality control testing according to package inserts

- Correcting problems discovered during quality control testing before testing patient samples

- Establishing policies for frequency of control testing

- Carefully following all test timing recommendations

- Interpreting test results using product insert information

- Recording test results according to policies and procedures

- Reporting test results to physicians in a timely manner

- Following package insert recommendations for follow-up or confirmatory testing

- Following OSHA regulations for biohazardous waste disposal

- Participating in quality assurance and assessment programs for every test that is performed

Transport Specimens Based on Handling Requirements (e.g., Temperature, Light, Time)

After ensuring patient safety and completing the venipuncture technique properly, the next important step for the phlebotomist is transporting the specimens in a timely manner to the testing laboratory, and abiding by any specific handling requirements for each ordered test.

Phlebotomists working in a hospital or large laboratory facility will have fewer handling issues to remember because the drop-off point is usually in the same building and often where you are assigned to work. Still, you may on occasion perform venipuncture procedures for tests that require special handling, such as placing the specimen in ice slurry for transport to the lab, or conversely, keeping the specimen at body temperature, or protecting it from light exposure. Examples of tests that require special handling include ammonia and lactic acid, which require that the blood tube sit in an ice slurry immediately after draw; cold agglutinins must be kept at body temperature (37° C); you must protect bilirubin and serum folate, which you can achieve by wrapping the blood tube in foil.

In tests that have a time element, phlebotomists like you must pay attention to the predraw requirements, which often include the patient taking a specific medication, or drinking a prepared liquid, such as for a glucose tolerance test. Other examples may include a 2-hr postprandial, which would require a fasting blood sugar followed by a blood sugar test at exactly 2 hr after the patient started eating her meal. Other timed tests include peak and trough values for antibiotics like gentamycin or vancomycin, which are drawn in relation to the administration of the antibiotics. Coordinate these phlebotomy procedures with the nursing staff to ensure accurate results.

Whether the tests you are collecting require specific timing, heat, cold, or protection from light, as the phlebotomist, your role in transporting specimens to the laboratory after collection is as important as the venipuncture in securing a high-quality test result.

Explain Nonblood, Specimen Collection Procedures to Patients

Physicians order tests on fecal (**stool**) specimens to detect parasites, micro-organisms that cause **enteric** disease, **occult blood**, and colorectal cancer. Often, these tests accompany blood work, and therefore, as a phlebotomist, you may need to explain the tests, and how to collect them, to your patients.

Instruct patients that fecal specimens are collected into wide-mouthed containers that have tight-fitting lids. If they are collecting the specimen at home, the patient must avoid getting any urine into the sample, because this can kill micro-organisms important to the identification of disease. After collection, clean the outside of the collection container thoroughly. Transport the specimen immediately to the laboratory, and maintain it at body temperature. For fecal occult blood testing, patients will collect small amounts of feces on special test cards over three separate days. For a fecal fat analysis, a 72-hr refrigerated stool specimen is needed.

Urine is the most common nonblood specimen in the clinical laboratory. Urine specimens should be between 12 mL and 50 mL. Label each specimen container with the patient's name as well as the date and time of collection. Labels must be placed on the containers themselves, not the caps. Record all medications the patient is taking on the laboratory requisition form as well as the patient's chart. Menstruating women should not undergo urine tests until their cycle is over.

Urine collection requires a wide-mouthed container. Cover the container with a lid, and keep in the refrigerator until testing or test immediately. There are several common types of urine specimens:

- **Random specimen** – This is the most common form, which can be taken at any time.

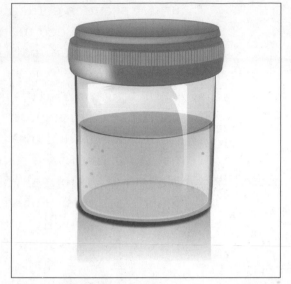

- **Clean-catch midstream specimen** – Instruct the patient to collect this after cleansing the genital area with soap and water or a prepackaged wipe. Physicians will order this test to diagnose urinary tract or kidney infections or to evaluate drug effectiveness. If a culture and sensitivity (C&S) test appears on the lab requisition, have the patient collect this type of specimen with minimal contamination. It is also important that the container be sterile. Provide antiseptic towelettes so the patient

Urine specimens require a wide-mouthed container with a lid.

can clean the perineal area (in females) or the penis (in males). Instruct patients to rinse away any soap residue because it can affect the specimen's pH. After cleansing the area, have the patient void some urine into the toilet as a discard amount, then collect the specimen, voiding into the container. After filling the container, the patient may void additional urine into the toilet. They will submit the closed container to the laboratory.

- **Timed specimen** – Patients will collect urine over a predetermined time period. Have the patient discard the first specimen in the period. After this, the patient will collect all urine within the specified time period. Physicians order these tests, including glucose tolerance tests, for a variety of reasons. Urine should not contact either stool or toilet paper. Instruct the patient to refrigerate the specimen until he delivers it to the physician's office or laboratory.

- 24-hour specimen – Sometimes, a physician will order a patient to collect urine output during a 24-hr period to test for substances released sporadically into the urine or to evaluate urine output. During this type of collection, patients must avoid bedpans, urinals, and toilet paper because they may retain the substances being tested, interfering with the testing. Instruct the patient to discard the first specimen. The patient will urinate into a small collection container, and pour this into a larger collection container. Have the patient clean the small container with soap and warm water between collections. Remind the patient to refrigerate the urine prior to delivery to the physician's office or laboratory if necessary.

- First-voided morning specimen – This is a specimen a patient collects in the morning immediately upon waking. The benefit of obtaining first-morning urine is that the concentrations of substances that collect overnight in urine are found in greater concentrations than specimens taken during the day. Use a urine specimen container or a clean, dry jar for collection. Physicians commonly order a first-voided morning specimen for pregnancy testing, culturing, and microscopic examination.

- Catheterization – This is the insertion of a sterile, flexible, narrow plastic tube (**catheter**) through the urethra into the bladder in order to withdraw urine. Catheterization allows the clinician to obtain a sterile urine specimen when a patient cannot void naturally, or to measure the amount of residual urine in the bladder after normal voiding. Physicians will sometimes order catheterization on female patients to prevent vaginal contamination of a specimen, or on infants for culture and sensitivity tests. Catheterization is not a routine specimen collection process because of the risk of infection.

- **Suprapubic** specimen – Physicians will sometimes order urine from a suprapubic tap. This involves the use of a sterile syringe with a needle that a physician inserts directly into the urinary bladder to aspirate urine for microbial analysis or cytology studies.

Semen collection requires the use of clean containers that are free of spermicides or detergents. The patient collects the semen himself and brings it immediately to the physician or laboratory. If using a condom for this purpose, it must be free of spermicides. DO NOT expose specimens to light or extreme temperatures. They must be kept as close to body temperature as possible. If you, as the phlebotomist, transport semen samples, wear gloves. Samples must reach the laboratory in less than 2 hr.

Sputum is mucus or phlegm that humans eject from the trachea and lungs through deep coughing. Collect sputum in a sterile container for microbiology specimens. When the collection is for a tuberculosis test, the container contains a poisonous preservative. Patients and phlebotomists must be very careful during collection and transportation of the specimen.

Handle Patient-Collected, Nonblood Specimens

In many settings, the phlebotomy team accepts and accessions, or checks in, all specimens that come into the laboratory for testing. Therefore, it is important for you to know how to properly handle and process these nonblood specimens.

Label every type of collection container with the patient's name, date and time of collection, and the specimen type.

When handling patient-collected, nonblood specimens, you must wear gloves. Proper handling is essential, and improper handling can affect the quality of the specimen. For example, components of urine change if the specimen stands at room temperature. Refrigerate urine specimens and process within 1 hr of collection. You may use evacuated transport tubes containing preservatives for transporting urine specimens to reference laboratories. To transfer the urine from the collection container to the transport container, use a pipette, or pour the urine into the tube after the stopper is removed. Preservatives in these tubes prevent bacterial overgrowth and stop changes in the urine that can affect test results.

When handling preserved specimens, the tubes may be kept at room temperature for up to 72 hr for **chemical reagent strip testing**. Tubes for culture and sensitivity tests may also be kept at room temperature for up to 72 hr. Complete the laboratory request forms for all specimens for transport to other sites for analysis. This form should include the patient's name, date, type of test ordered, ordering physician's name, the ICD-9-CM code used for diagnosis (if required), and a line where the physician may sign after reviewing the results. When sending specimens to the laboratory, use plastic **biohazard** bags with zipper seals. These bags feature an outside pocket into which you may place the laboratory request.

Avoid Preanalytical Errors When Collecting Blood Specimens

It is easy to miss errors in collection or handling unless there are obvious characteristics, such as hemolysis, clots, or underfilled tubes. These factors can cause inaccurate results. To avoid preanalytical errors when collecting blood specimens, do the following:

- Allow alcohol to fully dry prior to venipuncture.

- Use the appropriate gauge needle for the patient: nothing less than a 25-gauge needle to collect blood.

- Stop the draw if a hematoma forms.

- Avoid forceful squeezing or "milking" during dermal puncture.

- Avoid vigorous mixing of the collection tube.

- Avoid pushing on the plunger during a syringe transfer procedure so blood is not forced out.

- Gently handle specimens during transport.

- Avoid freezing or thawing specimens in transit.

- Make sure that the order of draw is correct.

- Mix each tube properly after removing from the tube holder.

- Transfer specimens promptly from syringes to evacuated tubes.

- Use tubes that have not expired.

- Purge the air out of winged infusion set needle tubing by using "discard tubes," especially when drawing a light blue top tube.

- Always remove tubes when blood reaches the fill level.

- Use proper technique to minimize clotting in dermal puncture sites.

- Use correct tubes for collection.

- Understand and interpret requisitions correctly.

- Properly protect light- and temperature-sensitive specimens.

- Avoid using alcohol as an antiseptic during collection when instructions say to do so.

- Centrifuge specimens correctly.

- Correctly and completely label all specimens.

Adhere to Chain-of-Custody Guidelines When Required

The process that maintains control of and accountability for each specimen from the time of collection to the time of disposal is called the **chain of custody**. The identity of every individual who has handled a specimen, and each time that the specimen transfers, must be documented by the chain-of-custody form. Chain-of-custody forms require the following components:

- The name and identifying information of the patient or subject from whom the specimen was collected

- The name of the person who obtained and processed the specimen

- The date, location, and signature of the person attesting that the specimen is the correct one and matches its documentation

- The signature and date from every person that had possession of the specimen for any amount of time, even for transport

In the case of a driving under the influence (DUI) charge, police may request blood alcohol levels. The person in question must consent to having the blood test performed and may refuse it. Written consent is required, and if a phlebotomist attempts to collect a specimen without it, she may be guilty of assault and battery. Additionally, without consent, the blood alcohol test will not be admissible in court. Because these specimens are often key evidence in legal cases, the phlebotomist must take great care during collection and closely monitor the chain of custody. Clean the site from which blood is taken with an appropriate antiseptic, such as chlorhexidine. Do not use alcohol for this purpose because it could lead to a false positive result. Also avoid iodine swabs because they contain alcohol.

Prepare Samples for Transportation to a Reference (Outside) Laboratory

When a facility does not conduct certain tests, you may need to prepare the samples for transportation to an outside laboratory known as a **reference laboratory**. If specimens are sent via the mail or express delivery services, they must fully comply with local, state, and federal laws that govern their special packaging and biohazard identification.

To prepare samples for transportation to a reference laboratory, package the specimens using the following:

- Original specimen tubes or plastic screw-cap transfer tubes

- Absorbent materials

- Watertight primary containers

- Watertight secondary containers (including resealable bags, plastic canisters, or foam boxes)

- Strong outer packaging (including fiberboard boxes or mailing tubes, wooden boxes, or rigid plastic containers)

- Coolants (ice packs or dry ice), if indicated

- Correct and complete shipping paperwork, including patient identification, specimen identification, and test information

To correctly prepare these samples, place the labeled specimen into a primary container, which is surrounded by absorbent material and usually located above any required coolants. All of these materials are contained within the secondary container. Specimen documentation is placed above the secondary container. Then the secondary container and documentation are placed inside the shipping container.

Coordinate Communication Between Nonlaboratory Personnel

Phlebotomists interact with many medical professionals, including physicians, nurses, laboratory technicians, respiratory technicians, and x-ray technicians. It is important to coordinate communication between nonlaboratory personnel regarding processing and collection, and to monitor and adjust according to best practices and patient needs.

Computerized programs now manage work flows and communications specific to each physician or provider of services. In addition to computer communications, effective communication involves using standard terminology and abbreviations, and proper documentation. Documentation can include recording contact notes on lab reports or lab logs.

In today's health care delivery system, computers and networks play key roles in the scheduling, managing and processing of patients, specimens, and clinical work flow. As a phlebotomist, you will need to become familiar with the software, communication methods, and processes within your organization. Software that supports the ordering, processing, and routing of specimens helps to streamline work flows that once were paper-intensive. Computer programs that link test results to physician or provider alerts depending on preset values contribute to an effective and efficient communication process. Each organization will establish policies and procedures for communications around specimen processing and collection.

Use Technology to Input and Retrieve Specimen Data

In the clinical laboratory, computer (and related) technology is used every day to input and retrieve specimen data. It allows the following:

- Entering lists of test requisitions

- Generating labels, schedules, and specimen collection lists

- Managing inventory

- Printing lists

- Record-keeping

- Reporting and storing test and quality control results

- Sending charges for procedures to the accounting office

- Sending test results to nursing stations and other locations

- Updating records of specimens that are already in the lab and in process (e.g., add-on tests)

As a phlebotomist, you may work with laboratory information systems, electronic medical records, and scheduling systems in your daily job tasks. Each organization's system and process will be unique. Your role as a phlebotomist will include learning the system, and using it in accordance with the policies and procedures set by the facility.

Report Critical Values for Point-of-Care Testing

Laboratory testing that is performed close to the site of patient care (such as at the patient bedside, or in the exam room of a physician office) is known as **point-of-care** testing. Clinical staff members often conduct point-of-care testing. A critical value is a test result that is significantly higher or lower than normal and may indicate a potential life-threatening situation for the patient. A phlebotomist performing point-of-care testing must be aware of the values that indicate a potential life-threatening or health-endangering situation. When a critical value occurs, report these results promptly and directly to the ordering provider. Not all laboratory values have a critical level, but each laboratory or facility will have a list of the tests for which you will need to monitor patient results for critical values. Learning the difference between an elevated or decreased value, and a critical value is important. Blood glucose level is a common point-of-care test. Diabetic patients will routinely have results outside the high limits of normal for a nondiabetic patient, but the results are "within normal limits" for them. As a phlebotomist, you need to know when a high result is "normal," or expected, for a patient due to her condition, and when to notify the physician.

Some phlebotomists keep an index card of critical values in their lab coat or phlebotomy tray until they learn them. The specific critical values may differ from facility to facility and may change over time. Become familiar with the general tests that physicians monitor for critical values, and learn the values for your organization.

Distribute Laboratory Results to Ordering Providers

Ordering providers receive laboratory results through verbal, telephone, written, or computer reports depending on the urgency of the values. Report critical results immediately with a telephone call, and document the report by obtaining the full name of the person receiving the results, and the date and time he took the information. Some offices print and mail routine results. You may e-mail or fax results to the ordering provider if appropriate secure transmission channels are in place. Since the implementation of the **meaningful use** incentive program that encourages physicians and other health care providers to adopt health information technology, physician offices using electronic medical records can now link with laboratories to receive patient results automatically by a **continuity of care document (CCD)**. When sharing verbal results, document the patient's name, identification number, the name of the person receiving the report, the date and time, the information, and the origination of the report or results. Information systems and networks allow for almost instant sharing of test results and reports. Printers generate hard copies of test results, which you may then fax or mail. Written and computerized reports are less prone to error than verbal or telephone reports of laboratory results. Regardless of the type of report, as a phlebotomist, you must maintain patient privacy and confidentiality.

Summary

The CLIA allows testing that involves lower complexity and/or minimum risk to patients in a patient's home or in a medical facility. If a laboratory has a certificate of waiver (for waived tests), it must submit to random inspections and investigation, as required by CLIA. Physicians order stool, urine, semen, and sputum samples for various tests, which you must adequately explain to patients. Proper handling of patient-collected, nonblood specimens is essential because improper handling can affect the quality of the specimen.

To prevent preanalytical errors when collecting blood specimens, the phlebotomist should avoid the following: forceful squeezing during dermal puncture, vigorous mixing of collection tubes, pushing on plungers during syringe transfer procedures, using alcohol during collection in certain instances, and leaving a tourniquet on too long during collection.

When you receive an order for blood alcohol, drug testing, and forensic testing, handle the documentation carefully to preserve the chain of custody for specimens. Shipments of specimens to reference laboratories must fully comply with laws that govern packaging and biohazard identification.

As a phlebotomist, you will interact with many other types of medical professionals. It is important that you coordinate communication between these individuals in order to reduce misunderstandings and errors. Computers and related technology help to improve communications and the quality of patient care. Point-of-care critical values must be reported immediately to the ordering provider. Written and electronic laboratory result reporting helps to reduce errors and increase quality of care. Always protect patient privacy and confidentiality regardless of the type of methods used for specimen collection, testing, and the reporting of results.

Drill Questions

1. Blood glucose, pregnancy, and fecal blood testing are examples of which of the following types of test?

    A. High-complexity tests
    B. Moderate-complexity tests
    C. Physician-performed microscopy tests
    D. Waived tests

2. Fecal specimen collection is used to detect which of the following?

    A. Urinary bladder cancer
    B. Colorectal cancer
    C. Lower esophageal cancer
    D. Diverticulosis

3. Which of the following types of urine collection is required for culture and sensitivity testing?

    A. 24-hour specimen
    B. First-voided morning specimen
    C. Clean-catch midstream specimen
    D. Timed specimen

4. For which of the following tests would a first-voided morning urine specimen be collected?

    A. Drug
    B. Alcohol
    C. Glucose
    D. Pregnancy

5. Patients and phlebotomists must be very careful during collection of sputum samples for a tuberculosis test for which of the following reasons?

    A. They are highly light- and temperature-sensitive.
    B. They may contain high levels of blood alcohol.
    C. The collection containers have a poisonous preservative inside them.
    D. The collection containers have a poisonous fungicide inside them.

6. Tubes needed for culture and sensitivity tests may be kept at room temperature for up to how many hours?

    A. 2
    B. 12
    C. 24
    D. 72

7. Sealed or locked specimen transfer bags are used as part of which of the following?

    A. Chain of custody
    B. Plasma thawing
    C. Centrifuging
    D. Chain of communication

8. Which of the following is required for all specimens shipped to a reference laboratory?

    A. Chain-of-custody form
    B. A warming pack
    C. Watertight secondary containers
    D. An ice pack

Drill Answers

1. Blood glucose, pregnancy, and fecal blood testing are examples of which of the following types of test?

    A. High-complexity tests
    B. Moderate-complexity tests
    C. Physician-performed microscopy tests
    D. Waived tests

    Waived tests are those that require a minimum of judgment and interpretation, including test kits approved for home use. They include blood glucose, pregnancy, and fecal blood tests. The other answer choices are incorrect because they all require various levels of medical training.

2. Fecal specimen collection is used to detect which of the following?

    A. Urinary bladder cancer
    B. Colorectal cancer
    C. Lower esophageal cancer
    D. Diverticulosis

    Fecal (stool) specimens are often collected to detect colorectal cancer. Urinary bladder cancer is confirmed by cystoscopy and biopsy. Lower esophageal cancer and diverticulosis can be detected by endoscopy.

3. Which of the following types of urine collection is required for culture and sensitivity testing?

    A. 24-hour specimen
    B. First-voided morning specimen
    C. Clean-catch midstream specimen
    D. Timed specimen

    A clean-catch midstream specimen is collected after the genital area is cleaned. It is often ordered to diagnose urinary tract infections or to evaluate drug effectiveness. This type of specimen is required for culture and sensitivity tests because it uses specimens that are free from contamination, in sterile containers. The other answer choices do not.

4. For which of the following tests would a first-voided morning urine specimen be collected?

    A. Drug
    B. Alcohol
    C. Glucose
    D. Pregnancy

    To help confirm pregnancy, a first-voided morning specimen is collected because of the high concentration of substances in the urine. Drug and alcohol tests may be inaccurate if the patient waits for 8 hr. Glucose tests are normally performed via routine or timed specimens.

5. Patients and phlebotomists must be very careful during collection of sputum samples for a tuberculosis test for which of the following reasons?

    A. They are highly light- and temperature-sensitive.
    B. They may contain high levels of blood alcohol.
    C. The collection containers have a poisonous preservative inside them.
    D. The collection containers have a poisonous fungicide inside them.

    Sputum may be tested for pathogenic organisms such as tuberculosis, and may be collected in containers that have a preservative for cytology testing. Because this preservative is poisonous, patients and phlebotomists must be very careful during collection. The other answer choices do not relate to sputum samples.

6. Tubes needed for culture and sensitivity tests may be kept at room temperature for up to how many hours?

    A. 2
    B. 12
    C. 24
    D. 72

    Tubes needed for culture and sensitivity tests may be kept at room temperature for up to 72 hr. This is also true for preserved urine specimens. The other answer choices are too short for exposure to room temperature for these specimens.

7. Sealed or locked specimen transfer bags are used as part of which of the following?

    A. Chain of custody
    B. Plasma thawing
    C. Centrifuging
    D. Chain of communication

    For chain of custody, specimens are placed into specimen transfer bags. These are sealed or locked until they are opened for specimen analysis. The seals on these bags ensure tamper-evident transfer. The other answer choices do not pertain to specimen transfer bags.

8. Which of the following is required for all specimens shipped to a reference laboratory?

    A. Chain-of-custody form
    B. A warming pack
    C. Watertight secondary containers
    D. An ice pack

    Watertight secondary containers include resealable bags, plastic canisters, and foam boxes. These are used, along with watertight primary containers and strong outer packaging, to transport samples to reference laboratories. Ice and warming packs may be necessary but are not always required. A chain-of-custody form may be necessary depending on the sample, but it is not required for all specimens.

Terms and Definitions

Biohazard – Anything that is a risk to organisms, such as ionizing radiation or harmful bacteria or viruses

Catheter – A hollow, flexible tube that can be inserted into a vessel or cavity of the body to withdraw fluids

Chain of custody – The chronological documentation (paper trail) showing the seizure, custody, control, transfer, analysis, and disposition of specimens that may be used as evidence

Chemical reagent strip testing – A method of urinalysis involving the use of plastic strips to which chemically specific reagent pads are affixed

Clean-catch midstream specimen – A method of urine collection that may be ordered to diagnose urinary tract infections or to evaluate the effectiveness of drug therapy

Continuity of care document (CCD) – A document that conforms to a standard, accepted format for electronically transmitting/sharing patient information securely and in a format that is easy to read and share among provider locations.

Enteric – Pertaining to the intestines

Meaningful use – A federal incentive program sponsored by the Centers for Medicare and Medicaid Services (CMS) that encourages physicians and hospitals to adopt health information technology solutions, such as electronic health record technology, and the transfer of electronic information between providers by giving financial awards for meeting specific criteria.

Occult blood – Blood that comes from a source that cannot be immediately determined, such as a peptic ulcer

Point of care – At or near the site of patient care

Quality control – A method of repeated assay of known standard materials and monitoring reaction parameters to ensure precision and accuracy

Random specimen – A single urine specimen taken at any time

Reagents – Chemical substances known to react in specific ways; reagents are used to detect or synthesize other substances in chemical reactions

Reference laboratory – A laboratory that is outside a patient care facility; usually, reference laboratories are able to perform many more types of testing than are available at the average hospital laboratory

Semen – The thick, whitish secretion of the male reproductive organs discharged from the urethra during ejaculation

Sputum – Material coughed up from the lungs and expectorated through the mouth

Stool – Also called feces; waste or excrement from the digestive tract that is formed in the intestine and expelled through the rectum

Suprapubic – Pertaining to a location above the symphysis pubis, which is the slightly movable interpubic joint of the pelvis, consisting of two pubic bones separated by a disk of fibrocartilage and connected by two ligaments

Timed specimen – Collected over a predetermined time period to obtain more specific information; such specimens are sometimes collected 2 hr after a meal to test for diabetes

Urine – The fluid secreted by the kidneys, transported by the ureters, stored in the bladder, and voided through the urethra

04 SAFETY AND COMPLIANCE CONSIDERATIONS

Learning Objectives
At the end of this chapter, you will be able to:

- *Adhere to regulations regarding workplace safety (e.g., OSHA, NIOSH).*

- *Adhere to regulations regarding operational standards (e.g., The Joint Commission, CLSI).*

- *Adhere to HIPAA regulations regarding protected health information (PHI).*

- *Follow exposure control plans in the event of occupational exposure.*

- *Follow transmission-based precautions (e.g., iatrogenic, airborne, droplet, contact, hospital-acquired infection).*

- *Wear personal protective equipment while following standard precautions (e.g., gloves, gowns, masks, shoe covers).*

- *Sanitize hands to prevent the spread of infections.*

- *Initiate first aid when necessary.*

- *Initiate CPR when necessary.*

Overview

Many different regulatory bodies control workplace safety, and ensure the compliance of employers in providing safe working environments. The Occupational Safety and Health Administration (OSHA) strictly regulates exposure to biologic hazards in the workplace. In addition, the Bloodborne Pathogens Standard requires implementation of work practice and engineering controls to prevent exposure incidents. One of the most effective means of preventing infection is proper hand hygiene. One of the most successful first aid measures is proper application of cardiopulmonary resuscitation (CPR). This technique can provide oxygen to the brain and prevent brain damage, as well enable a patient to survive cardiac or pulmonary arrest until advanced life support becomes available. The Joint Commission and the Clinical and Laboratory Standards Institute (CLSI) are responsible for the accreditation of various health care facilities. The creation of privacy and security laws affecting health care, such as HIPAA, works to improve efficiency while protecting patient privacy. HIPAA requires health care providers to maintain patient confidentiality at all times.

Adhere to Regulations Regarding Workplace Safety (e.g., OSHA, NIOSH)

Health care facilities must provide biologically safe working environments as set forth by the Occupational Safety and Health Administration (OSHA), accrediting agencies, the Centers for Disease Control and Prevention (CDC), and state regulatory agencies. OSHA, as a part of the Department of Labor, maintains regulatory standards directed at minimizing occupational exposure to hazardous chemicals in laboratories. These standards require chemical manufacturers to supply material safety data sheets (MSDSs) for their chemicals. Each MSDS bears a hazard warning label and lists information about a chemical, including protective measures that should be taken when working with the chemical. This information includes the chemical name, trade name, synonyms, manufacturer's name, address, emergency telephone number, and information about protective measures that should be taken when working with the chemical.

OSHA strictly regulates exposure to **biologic hazards**. Workplaces must have the Occupational Exposure to Bloodborne Pathogens program in place. According to OSHA, thousands of health care workers are infected with hepatitis B every year, making it the most commonly occurring laboratory-acquired infection. OSHA's **Bloodborne Pathogens Standard** covers all employees who may come in contact with blood and other infectious materials during their regular jobs. OSHA has regulations concerning hazards, including radioactive materials. Employers must maintain a written **exposure control plan** and document the destruction or removal of biohazardous waste.

The Bloodborne Pathogens Standard requires implementation of work practice and engineering controls to prevent exposure incidents, special training, availability, and use of personal protective equipment, medical surveillance, and the availability of the hepatitis B vaccination for all "at-risk" employees. Revised in 2001, the standard now has more complete definitions relating to engineering controls, new record-keeping requirements, an updated exposure control plan, and requests employee input about work practice and engineering controls selected. The term **decontamination** is used by OSHA to describe the use of physical or chemical means of removing, inactivating, or destroying blood-borne pathogens.

Follow Exposure Control Plans in the Event of an Occupational Exposure

Document all safety practices and precautions in the workplace's safety manual, and include clear explanations that describe the steps to take when a mishap occurs. Include evacuation plans as well as emergency numbers of area hospitals, fire, police, and security personnel, and post these near every phone. Documentation must exist for accidents (accident logs) in addition to instructions on how to correctly document accidents.

The National Institute for Occupational Safety and Health (NIOSH) has annually updated regulations regarding workplace safety that primarily include the handling and usage of sharps containers.

Sharps containers must:

- Be leak- and puncture-proof

- Be easy to identify and determine when they are full; this avoids overfilling and reduces the risk of injury

- Display a biohazard symbol

- Be stable to prevent slipping during use

Other NIOSH regulations require employers and health care employees to do the following:

- Implement the use of devices with safety features, and evaluate their use to determine which are most effective and acceptable.

- Set priorities and strategies for prevention by examining local and national information about risk factors for needle-stick injuries and successful intervention efforts.

- Modify work practices that pose a needle-stick injury hazard to make them safer.

- Promote safety awareness in the work environment.

- Use devices with safety features provided by the employer.

- Avoid recapping needles.

- Plan for safe handling and disposal before beginning any procedure using needles.

- Dispose of used needles promptly in appropriate sharps disposal containers.

- Report all needle stick and other sharps-related injuries promptly to ensure that employees receive appropriate follow-up care.

- Tell the employer about hazards from needles observed in the work environment.

Participate in blood-borne pathogen training, and follow recommended infection prevention practices, including hepatitis B vaccination. If you are exposed to blood or body fluids, immediately wash the area of the splash, needle stick, or cut with soap and water. If the exposure came through a splash, rinse the affected area with water. For a splash that lands in your eye, flush with sterile saline if available. Clean water is also acceptable for use in the case of eye contamination. It is important that you then report the incident to your supervisor and immediately seek a medical evaluation for the exposure. As in other non-routine situations, it is best to locate the resources you will need before an incident occurs. Know where the eye wash stations are located, and learn the procedures at your facility for reporting an exposure to blood or body fluids when on the job.

Adhere to Regulations Regarding Operational Standards

The Joint Commission accredits and certifies more than 19,000 health care organizations in the United States. It is an independent, nongovernmental, nonprofit organization with global recognition. The Joint Commission's operational standards focus on continual improvement of patient safety and quality of care. The Joint Commission updates the standards regularly to reflect the rapid advances in health care and medicine. There are more than 250 hospital accreditation standards, which address such areas as patient rights and education, infection control, medication management, medical errors, verification of staff competency, emergency preparedness, data collection, and operational improvement.

The Clinical and Laboratory Standards Institute (CLSI) provides voluntary consensus standards and guidelines for clinical laboratory professionals seeking to meet accreditation requirements. The CLSI guides the provision of better quality, highly effective service, focuses on assessment and improvement of quality control, improving patient care, reducing risks, and implementing time-saving methods and cost-cutting measures.

The CLSI's standards involve separate committees that focus on each laboratory area of development for these standards.

Adhere to HIPAA Regulations Regarding Protected Health Information (PHI)

The federal government's creation of laws around privacy and security in the health care setting serves to protect the privacy and security of patient information. Congressional representatives and legal and health care experts saw increasing challenges to protecting private information in a fast-growing technological environment. They enacted laws to standardize control over access to private health records. The primary goals of the Health Insurance Portability and Accountability Act (HIPAA) include the following:

- Improving the portability (ability to transmit and transfer information) and continuity of health care coverage

- Reducing abuse, fraud, and waste in health care delivery and insurance

- Promoting the use of medical savings accounts

- Improving access to long-term health care coverage and services

- Simplifying health insurance administration

HIPAA requires health care providers to maintain patient confidentiality at all times. It guides the use and disclosure of **protected health information** (PHI) by **covered entities**, such as hospitals and physicians. Health care providers must protect all health information, whether electronic, written, or verbal. Each patient has the right to be told about the potential use of PHI. HIPAA allows patients better access to their own health information while protecting it from disclosure to people or organizations that have no legitimate business need for the information.

Follow Transmission-Based Precautions (e.g., Iatrogenic, Airborne, Droplet, Contact)

Phlebotomists and other health care workers follow basic standard precautions when handling potentially infectious materials such as blood, urine, or other body fluids. There are cases, however, where you will need to observe additional precautions.

In any setting, if you are potentially infectious due to illness, it is in your patients' best interest for you to stay home until you are well. If this is not possible, consider wearing a mask to prevent coughing or sneezing from contaminating your patients through the spread of droplet contamination. Getting a cold or the flu from a health care worker is annoying at best, but for some patients, it can be deadly.

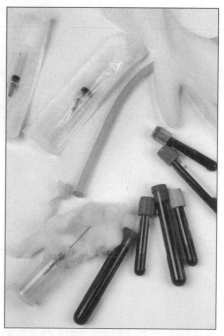

Protect your patients by using the right equipment.

Cancer patients, transplant recipients, and others who are immunocompromised (which means that their immune systems are not working up to full potential) are at a higher risk from health care workers who are ill. It is critical for you to observe proper technique to prevent the transmission of infectious agents, through hand hygiene, masks when appropriate, and attention to proper venipuncture technique.

In the inpatient environment, you may need to perform venipuncture procedures on patients who are in isolation due to their compromised immune status. Each facility will have specific policies and procedures for handling these patients, which may require that you wash your hands with a specific antibacterial agent and then don gloves, gown, and shoe covers before entering the patient room. Learn and comply with the requirements in your facility to protect yourself and your patients.

For patients in respiratory isolation, you may need to wear a specific respirator, such as an N-95 or N-99 respirator, which prevents very small airborne particles from entering your respiratory tract during normal breathing. When interacting with tuberculosis (TB) patients, wearing a respirator in addition to other personal protective equipment (PPE), such as gown and gloves, is a requirement. TB patients often stay in negative pressure rooms that restrict the airflow from the rest of the facility, and most hospitals have a respiratory isolation protocol in place that will dictate patient access procedures. Familiarize yourself with your facility's policies, and follow the required procedures at all times.

Patients who have infectious diseases that spread easily through contact are also placed in isolation. The most common infectious agents include methicillin-resistant *Staphylococcus aureus* (MRSA), vancomycin-resistant enterococcus (VRE), and *Clostridium difficile* (*C. diff*). Performing a venipuncture procedure on patients who have active infections like these requires PPE beyond gloves. In many facilities, a specific procedure for entering will be posted outside the room. This will include gloves, gown, mask, and shoe covers in many cases. *C. diff*, MRSA, and VRE are virulent and hard to treat, so preventing any contamination from leaving one patient's room on clothing, shoes, or skin is critical. Additionally, as a phlebotomist, you will not want to carry these pathogens home to your family. Familiarize yourself with the policy and procedure at your facility for managing contact with patients infected with these or other agents that require contact isolation.

Wear Personal Protective Equipment While Following Standard Precautions

For most venipuncture procedures in the outpatient and inpatient environment, you will follow the OSHA requirement, which mandates the use of latex or similar gloves. You will don additional PPE for patients whose condition is dangerous to health care workers, such as in cases of respiratory or contact isolation. You also will don additional PPE for patients who need protection from the potentially infectious agents that you, as a phlebotomist, may carry to in them.

Sanitize Hands to Prevent the Spread of Infection

Hand hygiene is the most effective means of preventing infection. Wash your hands when entering or leaving work areas, before and after patient procedures, after contact with any body fluid (even while wearing gloves), before and after eating, and before and after using the restroom.

When hands are not visibly soiled, you may use an alcohol-based hand sanitizer that has at least a 60% concentration of alcohol. Many hospitals, health care, and other facilities now provide wall-mounted or stand-alone dispensers to help promote regular attention to hand hygiene.

Initiate First Aid When Necessary

As a health care worker, you have a special responsibility to safeguard your patients' well-being. This means that you will need to learn and be able to apply basic first aid techniques if necessary for your patients.

In an inpatient setting, finding a patient in distress from a fall, an open wound, or chest pain would indicate a need to immediately contact the nurse or physician – whoever is closest. In outpatient settings, depending on the staff available, the best course of action will differ from setting to setting.

In a clinic or physician office setting, any patient condition that requires medical intervention should be brought to the attention of a physician or nurse on site. In an outpatient drawing station situation where you may be the only health care worker on site, you have an increased responsibility to prepare for medical emergencies so that you can provide basic first aid to your patients until additional help arrives.

Initiate CPR When Necessary

The efficiency, speed, and proper application of **cardiopulmonary resuscitation (CPR)** directly affects its success. In unconscious people, it is important to quickly determine the state of ventilation and circulation. Irreversible brain damage or death can result from a lack of oxygen that lasts for more than 4 to 6 min.

Once you identify a victim as unresponsive, call for help, and note the exact time of collapse or when you discovered the patient in this condition. Position the victim horizontally on a hard surface. For adults, the American Heart Association recommends "CAB," meaning that chest compressions are more important first, followed by airway assessment and rescue breathing. However, neonatal CPR is somewhat different (see http://www.heart.org/cpr).

Most cardiac arrest occurs in adults, and early chest compressions and defibrillation result in greater success. Continue CPR until the cardiopulmonary system is stable, advanced life support arrives, the patient is pronounced dead, or the rescuer cannot continue due to exhaustion. Resuscitation efforts include basic life support (using techniques and equipment that are immediately available), and advanced cardiac life support (involving drug therapy, cardiac monitoring, and other specialized techniques and equipment).

For adults, follow these steps to maintain basic life support:

- Determine if the patient is either not breathing or if breathing is impaired. Tap the victim's shoulder and ask, "Are you OK?" The airway is checked by tilting the victim's head back using the "head-tilt, chin-lift" maneuver. Breathing may be assessed by placing your ear near the patient's mouth while watching for movement of the patient's chest.

- If the patient is breathing and you do not suspect a spinal injury, place him in the **recovery position** (basically, lying on one side).

- Activate the emergency response system by calling 911 or the local emergency number, or have someone else call for you.

- Find a **defibrillator** (office defibrillators are portable, powered by either batteries or standard 110V current), and follow instructions found on the defibrillator.

- Begin CPR, pushing hard and fast, by placing the heel of one hand on the patient's sternum between the nipples and placing the other hand over the first, interlacing the fingers. Give at least 100 chest compressions per min, at least 1.5 to 2 inches deep. Make sure to allow the chest to fully recoil between compressions.

- If the patient starts moving, check for breathing. If this is adequate, place him in the recovery position, monitoring until a doctor or emergency medical services (EMS) arrives.

Chest compressions provide adequate blood circulation to the brain. Faster compressions (of adequate depth) result in a higher survival rate than slower, shallower compressions. Compressions create an increase in intrathoracic pressure, which then results in blood flow to the brain and other organs.

Note: The "adult chain of survival," in summary, is as follows:

- Immediate recognition of cardiac arrest, then activation of the emergency response system.

- Early cardiopulmonary resuscitation with emphases on chest compressions.

- Rapid defibrillation.

- Effective advanced life support.

Summary

Organizations like OSHA and NIOSH regulate workplace safety. There are hundreds of regulations in place to ensure safety in many types of workplaces. Organizations including the Joint Commission and CLSI set operational standards for hospitals and laboratories. Adherence to these standards helps keep both employees and employers safe. Protected health information is patient information that falls under the regulations of HIPAA. This legislation was created to improve overall health care practices in order to better protect patient information, and to increase speed and accuracy of activities in order to increase effectiveness and save time and money. Unresponsive individuals may require cardiopulmonary resuscitation (CPR). The most important aspect of CPR is chest compressions because these help to circulate blood to the brain regardless of the patient's ability to breathe normally. When performing CPR, be sure to alert the emergency response system, usually by calling 911, or having someone else do so. Time is of the essence because irreversible brain damage will occur if CPR is not performed correctly, or not performed quickly enough.

Drill Questions

1. Protective measures that should be taken when working with a chemical will be found listed in the chemical's

   A. material safety data sheet.
   B. exposure control plan.
   C. Bloodborne Pathogens Standard.
   D. hazard communication plan.

2. Which of the following is the most commonly occurring laboratory-acquired infection?

   A. Pneumonia
   B. Hepatitis B
   C. Human immunodeficiency virus
   D. Meningitis

3. A written exposure control plan must be maintained by which of the following?

   A. Practitioner
   B. Insurer
   C. Phlebotomist
   D. Employer

4. Operational standards are established by which of the following agencies?

   A. CDC
   B. CLSI
   C. CLIAC
   D. CLIA

5. Under which of the following circumstances should you place a patient into the recovery position?

   A. If the patient is not breathing and there is no pulse
   B. If the patient has not been breathing for at least 10 min
   C. If the patient is breathing and you do not suspect a spinal injury
   D. If the patient is breathing and you suspect a spinal injury

Drill Answers

1. Protective measures that should be taken when working with a chemical will be found listed in the chemical's

   A. material safety data sheet.
   B. exposure control plan.
   C. Bloodborne Pathogens Standard.
   D. hazard communication plan.

   Material safety data sheets list protective measures that should be taken when working with chemicals. Exposure control plans are designed to lower risks for exposure to various materials. The Bloodborne Pathogens Standard protects personnel who may face potential blood-borne pathogen exposure at work. The hazard communication plan is a system of notifying personnel of hazards by applying warning labels about substances being used in the workplace.

2. Which of the following is the most commonly occurring laboratory-acquired infection?

   A. Pneumonia
   B. Hepatitis B
   C. Human immunodeficiency virus
   D. Meningitis

   Hepatitis B is the most commonly occurring laboratory-acquired infection. The next most common of the given choices is human immunodeficiency virus. Pneumonia and meningitis are not commonly acquired in the laboratory.

3. A written exposure control plan must be maintained by which of the following?

   A. Practitioner
   B. Insurer
   C. Phlebotomist
   D. Employer

   The employer must maintain a written exposure plan. The phlebotomist may report to it but does not maintain it. The insurer and practitioner generally have nothing to do with the written exposure plan.

4. Operational standards are established by which of the following agencies?

    A. CDC
    B. CLSI
    C. CLIAC
    D. CLIA

    CLSI and the Joint Commission establish operational standards. CDC investigates disease outbreaks. CLIAC develops quality assurance practices. CLIA is the agency that sets standards for laboratories.

5. Under which of the following circumstances should you place a patient into the recovery position?

    A. If the patient is not breathing and there is no pulse
    B. If the patient has not been breathing for at least 10 min
    C. If the patient is breathing and you do not suspect a spinal injury
    D. If the patient is breathing and you suspect a spinal injury

    If the patient is breathing and you do not suspect a spinal injury, you should place the patient into the recovery position. The patient should then be monitored until a doctor or EMS arrives.

Terms and Definitions

Biologic hazards – Also called biohazards; any risks to organisms, including ionizing radiation and harmful bacteria or viruses; any conditions or phenomena that increase the probability of harm

Bloodborne Pathogens Standard – An OSHA-mandated set of requirements concerning protection against pathogenic micro-organisms that are transmitted via human blood and cause disease in humans; these pathogens include hepatitis B virus and human immunodeficiency virus

Cardiopulmonary resuscitation (CPR) – A basic emergency procedure for life support is used in cases of cardiac arrest to establish effective circulation and ventilation in order to prevent irreversible cerebral damage resulting from anoxia

Covered entities – Those that must comply with HIPAA and provide health care services regularly, including health plans, health care clearinghouses, and health care providers who transmit any health information in electronic form

Decontamination – The process of removing foreign material such as blood, body fluids, or radioactivity; it does not eliminate micro-organisms but is a necessary step preceding disinfection or sterilization

Defibrillator – A device that delivers an electrical shock at a preset voltage to the myocardium; used for restoring the normal cardiac rhythm and rate when the heart has stopped beating, or is fibrillating

Exposure control plan – An OSHA-compliant plan that explains ways to minimize or eliminate exposure of humans to blood-borne pathogens; in general, it should include its date of development, scope of information, universal precautions, engineering and work practice controls, personal protective equipment, and cover housekeeping, waste disposal, laundry, vaccinations with follow-up evaluations, communication, training, and first aid

Protected health information – As defined by HIPAA, any information, whether oral or recorded in any form, that is created or received by a health care provider; also relates to the past, present, or future physical or mental health or condition of an individual, the provision of health care to an individual, or the payment for the provision of health care to an individual.

Recovery position – One of a series of variations on a lateral recumbent or three-quarters prone position of the body, into which an unconscious, but breathing, casualty can be placed as part of first aid treatment

Anatomy and Physiology

The patient, Mrs. Susan Smith, is a 79-year-old woman who is small in stature and very thin. Her physician has ordered two laboratory tests for her: a complete blood count (CBC), a test that measures hemoglobin concentration, hematocrit, the red blood cell count, several specific aspects of the red blood cells (e.g., amount of hemoglobin in an average red blood cell), the white blood cell count and the white blood cell differential, and the platelet count; and an International Normalized Ratio (INR), a test that measures the ability of the blood to clot.

The patient is sitting down in the laboratory testing area; the time is 9 a.m. The phlebotomy technician enters the room, identifies himself (using his first name only), identifies himself as the phlebotomy technician, and informs the patient that he will be drawing her blood. The technician asks the patient to identify herself by name, asks her to tell him her date of birth and the last four digits of her Social Security number, and checks the patient's wrist band to see if the information she gave was correct. Except for checking the patient's wrist band, the technician did not make eye contact with the patient during this time; he had been reading the laboratory order forms on a computer. Mrs. Smith is visibly anxious; she shifts nervously in the chair, checks her watch several times, and constantly crosses and uncrosses her legs.

The technician gathers a winged infusion set (aka Butterfly needle), a tourniquet, an isopropyl alcohol swab, a small adhesive bandage, a 1-inch-by-1-inch gauze pad, and a lavender top collection tube and a blue top collection tube.

After gathering the supplies, he washes his hands, puts on latex disposable gloves, and then asks the patient which arm she has prefers to be used; she chooses her left arm. He places her arm on the arm of the chair, supporting it with a pad. He visually identifies and palpates the median antecubital vein and then places the tourniquet around her arm; after the tourniquet is in place, he asks her if it is too tight. He cleans the skin over the vein with the isopropyl alcohol swab, informs the patient that she will feel a slight sensation of pain, and then performs the venipuncture. A few seconds after inserting the needle, the technician releases the tourniquet. Again, during the procedure the phlebotomy technician did not make eye contact with the patient, he does not speak to her, and while performing the venipuncture he does not a) ask her how she is feeling or, b) look at her to see if she is okay.

Mrs. Smith had been nervous before the procedure, and after the needle was inserted she begins to sweat and feel dizzy, and she becomes very pale. As the technician withdraws the needle and places the gauze pad on the site of the venipuncture, Mrs. Smith suddenly loses conscious and falls forward out of the chair and on to the floor and strikes her head. The technician lifts her up, places her back in the chair, and when she wakes up, he offers her some water.

1. Why was Mrs. Smith at risk for fainting?

   A. She was actively bleeding.
   B. The ambient temperature was very hot.
   C. She had a heart attack.
   D. She is a thin woman of small stature.

2. What other factor directly contributed to this episode of fainting?

   A. Lack of communication
   B. High level of stress
   C. Improper venipuncture technique
   D. The time of day

3. The average woman typically has a blood pressure that

   A. is lower than the blood pressure of the average man.
   B. is higher than the blood pressure of the average man.
   C. is no different than the blood pressure of the average man.
   D. fluctuates more than the blood pressure of the average man.

4. What part of the patient care process did the technician fail to perform?

   A. Standard precautions
   B. Identifying the patient
   C. Patient assessment
   D. The venipuncture procedure

5. What could the technician have done to predict the risk of fainting?

   A. He could have used verbal and non-verbal communication.
   B. He could have allowed the patient more time before the venipuncture.
   C. He could have told the patient he had many years of experience.
   D. He could have asked her if she had ever had an episode of fainting.

Anatomy and Physiology: Answers

1. Why was Mrs. Smith at risk for fainting?

    A. She was actively bleeding.
    B. The ambient temperature was very hot.
    C. She had a heart attack.
    D. She is a thin woman of small stature.

Women typically have lower blood pressure then men, and this is especially true for women who are thin and of small stature. It is possible that the patient was actively bleeding, but there was no evidence of this, and it is not something that the technician could have discerned by an assessment. High ambient temperatures can cause fainting, but laboratories are air conditioned. A heart attack can cause loss of consciousness, but again there was no evidence the patient was suffering a heart attack, and the phlebotomy technician could not have determined whether a heart attack was occurring by a simple verbal and visual assessment.

2. What other factor directly contributed to this episode of fainting?

    A. Lack of communication
    B. High level of stress
    C. Improper venipuncture technique
    D. The time of day

A high level of stress is a common cause of fainting. The phlebotomy technician did not predict the risk of fainting or notice it was possible because of a lack of communication, but this was not a direct cause of the loss of consciousness. The venipuncture was performed correctly, and the time of day would not be a direct cause of fainting.

3. The average woman typically has a blood pressure that

    A. is lower than the blood pressure of the average man.
    B. is higher than the blood pressure of the average man.
    C. is no different than the blood pressure of the average man.
    D. fluctuates more than the blood pressure of the average man.

The average woman typically has a blood pressure that is lower than the blood pressure of the average man. There is no difference between the sexes in fluctuations of blood pressure.

4. What part of the patient care process did the technician fail to perform?

    A. Standard precautions
    B. Identifying the patient
    C. Patient assessment
    D. The venipuncture procedure

Standard precautions, patient identification, and the venipuncture procedure were all performed properly. However, the technician never made assessments to see whether the patient could tolerate the venipuncture or whether she was tolerating the venipuncture.

5. What could the technician have done to predict the risk of fainting?

    A. He could have used verbal and non-verbal communication.
    B. He could have allowed the patient more time before the venipuncture.
    C. He could have told the patient he had many years of experience.
    D. He could have asked her if she had ever had an episode of fainting.

The phlebotomy technician did not ask the patient about her condition before and during the venipuncture, and he did not visually check her condition during the procedure; doing so would not have prevented the episode of fainting, but it would have helped the technician be prepared for that possibility and could prevent possible injury from a fall. Allowing the patient more time prior to the procedure and informing the patient of the technician's experience and competence may help a patient's comfort level, but probably not in this case. Asking about previous episodes of fainting is a very good idea, but in this case it was obvious that the patient was at risk for fainting at that time.

Patient Care

Mr. Watson is an 83-year-old man who recently had a stroke and has a history of kidney failure. He recovered from his stroke and is oriented, ambulatory, and can speak clearly (his ability to speak was briefly lost after the stroke). He is currently taking aspirin and warfarin in order to prevent another stroke. He has come to the laboratory for two blood tests, an INR and a partial thromboplastin time (PT); the PT determines the ability of the blood to clot.

The patient is the only person in the waiting room, and there is only one chart in the active case rack. The phlebotomy technician picks up the chart, briefly reads it, and then walks into the waiting room and says, "Are you Mr. Watson?" The patient does not answer; he simply stands up and then follows the technician into the testing area; she does not turn around to see if he is following her, she simply assumes that he is. She directs the patient to sit down – points to a chair – and asks him if his birthday is the birthdate on the chart. The patient says yes, and the technician begins to prepare for the venipuncture procedure.

The technician gathers a winged infusion set, an isopropyl alcohol swab, a small adhesive bandage, a 1-inch-by-1-inch gauze pad, a tourniquet, and two blue top blood collection tubes. She washes her hands and then puts on a pair of latex disposable gloves. Because the technician is left-handed, she asks the patient to roll up his sleeve and extend his left arm. She places the tourniquet on the patient's arm and then visually assesses and then palpates the median antecubital vein. She cleans the skin over the area where she will perform the venipuncture and then inserts the needle. A few seconds after inserting the needle the technician releases the tourniquet. She looks up briefly to see if the patient is comfortable, and after the second collection tube is filled, she withdraws the needle.

The technician places the gauze pad over the venipuncture site and applies pressure for approximately five seconds. She leaves the gauze in place, covers it snugly with the adhesive bandage, and then tells the patient, "Thank you, Mr. Watson, you are all finished." The patient stands up and exits the testing area.

1. In order to properly identify a patient, a phlebotomy technician must ask the patient

   A. to state his name.
   B. if the date of birth on the chart is correct.
   C. the name of his physician.
   D. if he is scheduled for an INR and a PT.

2. Another method for properly identifying a patient is

    A. asking the patient to state his telephone number.
    B. checking the patient's wrist band.
    C. asking another phlebotomy technician if he remembers the patient.
    D. checking this patient to see if he has a dialysis shunt in his arm.

3. Knowing the patient had a stroke and seeing he is an older adult, the technician should

    A. speak very loudly and clearly.
    B. check the patient's blood pressure.
    C. ask the patient if he needs assistance with walking.
    D. assume the patient will be confused.

4. If a patient is taking aspirin or warfarin

    A. the technician should not put pressure on the venipuncture.
    B. an extra gauze pad should be placed on the venipuncture site.
    C. the technician should leave the tourniquet on during the entire procedure.
    D. pressure on the venipuncture site should be applied for longer than usual.

5. If a patient is taking any drug that decreases the ability of the blood to clot, the patient should

    A. be advised to not exercise for 24 hours after venipuncture.
    B. be advised to return if there is excessive bruising.
    C. be advised to skip the next dose of medication.
    D. be advised to drink extra fluids after the venipuncture.

Patient Care: Answers

1. In order to properly identify a patient, a phlebotomy technician must ask the patient

   A. to state his name.
   B. if the date of birth on the chart is correct.
   C. the name of his physician.
   D. if he is scheduled for an INR and a PT.

   One of the methods for properly identifying patients is to ask the patient to state his/her name. Asking the patient if a particular date of birth is correct can cause errors; the patient may not hear you correctly or may be confused and answer incorrectly. Asking a patient the name of the treating physician or asking the patient what test has been scheduled also can cause errors. Physicians obviously care for many patients, and a phlebotomy technician may care for five patients in a row who are all scheduled for the same test.

2. Another method for properly identifying a patient is

   A. asking the patient to state his telephone number.
   B. checking the patient's wristband.
   C. asking another phlebotomy technician if he remembers the patient.
   D. checking this patient to see if he has a dialysis shunt in his arm.

   Checking the patient's wristband is a useful method for properly identifying patients, but it should not be used alone; the wristband may have been put on the wrong patient. Asking the patient if information such as a telephone number is correct is unsafe, as is depending on another technician's memory. It is certainly possible that there could be more than one patient with a dialysis shunt who has arrived for blood tests.

3. Knowing the patient had a stroke and seeing he is an older adult, the technician should

   A. speak very loudly and clearly.
   B. check the patient's blood pressure.
   C. ask the patient if he needs assistance with walking.
   D. assume the patient will be confused.

   People who have had a stroke may have difficulty walking because a stroke can cause permanent brain damage. In addition, it is a good practice to make sure that all patients, regardless of their age or medical history, can ambulate safely. Hearing can be affected by a stroke, but it is insensitive to assume this and speak too loudly; start with a normal tone and volume and adjust as needed. Phlebotomy technicians do not check blood pressures, and not all patients who have had a stroke will be confused, so it is insensitive to assume this.

4. If a patient is taking aspirin or warfarin

    A. the technician should not put pressure on the venipuncture.
    B. an extra gauze pad should be placed on the venipuncture site.
    C. the technician should leave the tourniquet on during the entire procedure.
    D. pressure on the venipuncture site should be applied for longer than usual.

If the patient is taking aspirin or warfarin, the phlebotomy technician must apply pressure to the venipuncture site for longer than the normal time; each laboratory, hospital, etc., should have a protocol that specifies how long to apply pressure. Pressure should be applied to all venipuncture sites, and an extra gauze pad would not prevent excessive bleeding in patients taking anticoagulants drugs. A tourniquet should never be left on during the entire time of a venipuncture; this can cause hemoconcentration and excessive bleeding and/or bruising, and this is especially true in patients taking anticoagulants drugs.

5. If a patient is taking any drug that decreases the ability of the blood to clot, the patient should

    A. be advised to not exercise for 24 hours after venipuncture.
    B. be advised to return if there is excessive bruising.
    C. be advised to skip the next dose of medication.
    D. be advised to drink extra fluids after the venipuncture.

Patients who take anticoagulant drugs are at risk for excessive bleeding after venipuncture, and this can be uncomfortable and potentially harmful. There is no need for the patient to avoid exercise after a venipuncture unless the exercise may cause blunt trauma or excessive pressure to the venipuncture area. Only a physician can advise a patient to change his medication regimen, and there is no need for extra fluids after a venipuncture; these patients are at risk because of medications they take, and extra fluids would not increase or decrease the effects of these drugs.

The Phlebotomy Procedure

The patient, Angela Jones, is a 45-year-old woman who has come to the outpatient laboratory for a CBC, an INR, and serum electrolytes. The patient is HIV positive and is currently using the highly active antiretroviral treatment (HAART) drug regimen.

The patient is in the waiting room, and when the phlebotomy technician calls her name, she stands up. The technician makes sure the patient can ambulate safely, brings her into the testing area, and asks her to sit down.

After the patient has been seated, the phlebotomy technician identifies herself by first name only, identifies herself as the phlebotomy technician, and explains to the patient what will happen. The phlebotomy technician asks the patient to state her name, her birth date, and the last four digits of her Social Security number. The technician confirms that all of the given information is identical to what is on the patient's chart and checks the patient's wrist band, as well. The phlebotomy technician spends a minute or two reading the patient's chart and then asks the patient how long she has been using the HAART regimen, how well the medications are working, and if she has an active case of AIDS.

The technician gathers a winged infusion set, an isopropyl alcohol swab, a bottle of povidine-iodine, a small adhesive bandage, a 1-inch-by-1-inch gauze pad, a tourniquet, a blue top collection tube, a red top collection tube, and a lavender top collection tube. After that she puts on disposable gloves, a disposable face mask, and a disposable gown. She asks the patient which arm she would prefer for the venipuncture – the patient says she does not care – visually inspects and palpates the median antecubital vein, and then puts a tourniquet on the patient's arm, asking the patient if the tourniquet is too tight; the patient says no. The selected site is cleaned, first with the povidine-iodine and then with the isopropyl alcohol swab.

After asking the patient if she has any questions or worries about the procedure and warning the patient that the procedure causes slight pain, the phlebotomy technician performs the venipuncture. The first tube – the lavender top – is attached to the infusion set, and after five seconds, the tourniquet is released. After the lavender top tube is filled, the red top tube is attached and filled and then the blue top tube is attached and filled. Several times during the procedure the phlebotomist asks the patient how she is feeling, and the phlebotomist also looks to see if the patient is pale or sweaty.

After the last tube is filled, the technician asks the patient to place a gauze pad over the needle, and then the technician removes the needle. The technician asks the patient to put pressure on the venipuncture site. The technician tells the patient that she would do it herself, but "I'm worried you might bleed on me." The technician places the blood tubes in a heavy plastic bag and places a sticky label on the outside of the bag; the label has the patient's identifying information. She places the adhesive bandage over the gauze pad and leaves the room.

1. Standard precautions involve

    A. handwashing for the phlebotomist and the patient.
    B. treating all body fluids as if they were infected.
    C. asking the patient if she has any infectious diseases.
    D. wearing a disposable mask.

2. Povidine-iodine should be used for blood specimen collection

    A. when collecting blood cultures.
    B. if the patient is infected with HIV.
    C. if more than four collection tubes will be needed.
    D. when the patient is less than 16 years of age.

3. Handwashing should done before performing venipuncture

    A. if the patient has an infectious disease
    B. if the phlebotomist has an infectious disease.
    C. in every situation.
    D. in conjunction with the use of a mask and gown.

4. It is important to correctly perform the order of the draw because

    A. the correct order of the draw is more comfortable for the patient.
    B. an incorrect order of the draw requires a greater volume of blood.
    C. the correct order of the draw can be performed more quickly.
    D. an incorrect order of the draw can affect the accuracy of the tests.

5. Phlebotomy technicians should not ask about a patient's HIV status because

    A. the information isn't needed to perform care or prevent disease transmission.
    B. asking a patient might make her uncomfortable.
    C. this information should only be discussed with a physician.
    D. asking a patient about HIV status is always a HIPAA violation.

The Phlebotomy Procedure: Answers

1. Standard precautions involve

   A. handwashing for the phlebotomist and the patient.
   B. treating all body fluids as if they were infected.
   C. asking the patient if she has any infectious diseases.
   D. wearing a disposable mask.

   Standard precautions require health care personnel to treat all body fluids as if they were infected and to use the appropriate barrier equipment, depending on the situation. Patients do not need to wash their hands before a procedure because they are not at any great risk for infection from a venipuncture. If standard precautions are used, there is no need for health care personnel to ask patients whether they have an infectious disease. Standard precautions, if properly used, will be sufficient protection for any patient care situation. A disposable mask is used only if the patient has an infectious disease that is transmitted by such functions as breathing or coughing, and almost invariably these patients are easily and rapidly identified.

2. Povidine-iodine should be used for blood specimen collection

   A. when collecting blood cultures.
   B. if the patient is infected with HIV.
   C. if more than four collection tubes will be needed.
   D. when the patient is less than 16 years of age.

   Povidine-iodine or some type of iodine solution is used to clean the venipuncture site when collecting blood cultures. The solution is needed because the blood samples are being checked for the presence of bacteria, etc., and it is important to make sure the blood specimens will not be cross-contaminated with normal skin flora. There is no need to use anything other than isopropyl alcohol when collecting blood from patients infected with HIV or patients younger than age 16. The number of collection tubes needed would not affect the type of skin preparation that is needed for a venipuncture.

3. Handwashing should done before performing venipuncture

   A. if the patient has an infectious disease
   B. if the phlebotomist has an infectious disease.
   C. in every situation.
   D. in conjunction with the use of a mask and gown.

Standard precautions require that handwashing should be done before any patient contact and before performing any procedure, regardless of the patient's condition or the phlebotomy technician's state of health. A disposable mask and a gown are not needed for a routine venipuncture.

4. It is important to correctly perform the order of the draw because

   A. the correct order of the draw is more comfortable for the patient.
   B. an incorrect order of the draw requires a greater volume of blood.
   C. the correct order of the draw can be performed more quickly.
   D. an incorrect order of the draw can affect the accuracy of the tests.

Performing the order of the draw incorrectly can affect the accuracy of test results by introducing additives found in one tube into another. The correct order of the draw has no effect at all on patient comfort, the volume of blood that is needed for a venipuncture, or the speed with which the venipuncture can be completed.

5. Phlebotomy technicians should not ask about a patient's HIV status because

   A. the information isn't needed to perform care or prevent disease transmission.
   B. asking a patient might make her uncomfortable.
   C. this information should only be discussed with a physician.
   D. asking a patient about HIV status is always a HIPAA violation.

If the phlebotomy technician uses standard precautions, she will be protected from disease transmission, so it is not necessary to ask patients about their HIV status. It is true that asking a patient about her HIV status could make the patient uncomfortable, but even more important, the phlebotomist does not need to know. Other people aside from physicians can ask about HIV status, and although in many circumstances asking about HIV status would be a HIPAA violation (Note: HIPAA is a set of government regulations that protect patient privacy), there are exceptions.

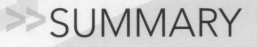

SUMMARY

This guide covered anatomy and physiology, the phlebotomy process, and patient care, as well as offering case studies to help you put teaching into action.

Earning the CPT certification demonstrates your commitment to excellence in the field, and is evidence of your desire to perform your duties as a phlebotomy technician in a professional manner. The CPT certification makes you a valuable member of the health care team and enables you to perform many vital tasks, including the invasive venipuncture procedure. Not only does certification demonstrate a high level of competency in CPT task performance, it also differentiates you from others who lack certification, enabling you to secure a job more easily and earn higher wages.

The information in this study guide prepares you for the CPT certification exam, as well as teaches you the information and knowledge you need to correctly, efficiently, and safely act in your role as a phlebotomy technician. This study guide presents information in six distinct sections, including an introduction; chapters on patient preparation, collection techniques, processing, and safety and compliance guidelines; three case studies; and this summary.

In the introduction, you learn all about the CPT certification exam, including its content and structure. Understanding the basics of the exam enables you to anticipate the types of questions you will encounter, and helps you achieve the highest possible score. Remember, the topics covered on the exam are anatomy and physiology; the phlebotomy procedure; professional behavior and communication; ethical and legal issues; and safety and infection control.

Chapter 1 provides you with an understanding of the basic patient preparation necessary prior to performing a phlebotomy procedure. Learning these steps is critical to becoming a CPT, and they give you a solid beginning on which to build your knowledge in the subsequent chapters.

Chapter 2 prepares you for basic blood collection through venipuncture and dermal punctures of the finger or heel. You will learn the proper techniques for safely and correctly obtaining quality specimens from patients who need testing performed. Accurately collecting specimens helps physicians and nurses provide the best care for patients. The CPT contributes to high quality health care delivery when performing duties in a safe and accurate manner. Chapter 2 also reviews cases of special collections. In some cases, the CPT will need to collect special types of specimens to meet patient needs. This chapter reviews the most common special collection practices and prepares you to safely and appropriately collect and process them.

Next, Chapter 3 reviews the many tasks of processing patient specimens after collection. After proper collection, careful handling and processing are most important to ensuring that the test results are timely and accurate and serve the best interest of the patients.

Chapter 4 reviews important safety and compliance guidelines when working with patients, their protected health information, and potentially infectious materials. CPTs must learn to work safely, protecting the health and safety or their patients, as well as themselves and fellow health care workers. They must follow laws and regulations in place to protect patients' privacy and the security of patient information, and to remain ready to assist when patient emergencies arise.

You represent the future of health care. Continually remain committed to keeping up with changes in the health care system. Also, consistently strive for a greater awareness of others, and how to best serve as a member of the health care team. Use the skills you acquire from this study guide to help yourself, and other CPTs succeed. Certified CPTs – like you – are valued members of the health care field.

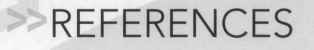

>>REFERENCES

Siegel, J.D., Rhinehart, E., Jackson, M., Chiarello, L. (2007). 2007 Guideline for Isolation Precautions: Preventing Transmission of Infectious Agents in Healthcare Settings. Retrieved from http://www.cdc.gov/hicpac/pdf/isolation/Isolation2007.pdf

Galena, H. J. (1992). Complications occurring from diagnostic venipuncture. *Journal of Family Practice, 34*(5), 582-584.

Garza, D., Becan-McBride, K. (2010). *Phlebotomy handbook* (8th ed.). Upper Saddle River, NJ: Pearson Education, Inc.

McCall, R. E. (2011). *Phlebotomy Essentials*. Philadelphia, PA: Lippincott, Williams & Wilkins.

National Committee for Clinical Laboratory Standards. (2007). Procedures for the collection of Diagnostic Blood Specimens by Venipuncture. Approved Standard H3-A6, Wayne, PA; 2003. Retrieved from http://www.clsi.org/source/orders/free/H3-a6.pdf

Occupational Safety and Health Administration. OSHA's Bloodborne Pathogens Standard. Retrieved from http://www.osha.gov/OshDoc/data_BloodborneFacts/bbfact01.pdf

Perspectives in Disease Prevention and Health Promotion Update: Universal Precautions for Prevention of Transmission of Human Immunodeficiency Virus, Hepatitis B Virus, and Other Bloodborne Pathogens in Health-Care Settings. *MMWR 37*(24), 377-388. Retrieved from http://www.cdc.gov/mmwr/preview/mmwrhtml/00000039.htm

Scales, K. (2008). A practical guide to venipuncture and blood sampling. *Nursing Standard, 22*(29), 29-36.

Vedder, T. G. (2011). *Heel Sticks*. Retrieved from http://emedicine.medscape.com/article/1413486-overview